HYGGE

The Danish Art of Happiness

By

Marie Tourell Søderberg

In collaboration with

Kathrine Højte Lynggaard

MICHAEL JOSEPH

an imprint of

PENGUIN BOOKS

MICHAEL JOSEPH

UK | USA | Canada | Ireland | Australia
India | New Zealand | South Africa

Michael Joseph is part of the Penguin Random House group of companies
whose addresses can be found at global.penguinrandomhouse.com.

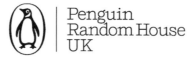

Penguin
Random House
UK

First published 2016
006

Copyright © Marie Tourell Søderberg, 2016

The moral right of the author has been asserted

Set in Bodoni and Futura
Design by Couper Street Type Co.
Printed in Italy by LEGO

A CIP catalogue record for this book is available from the British Library

ISBN: 978–0–718–18533–6

www.greenpenguin.co.uk

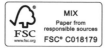

CONTENTS

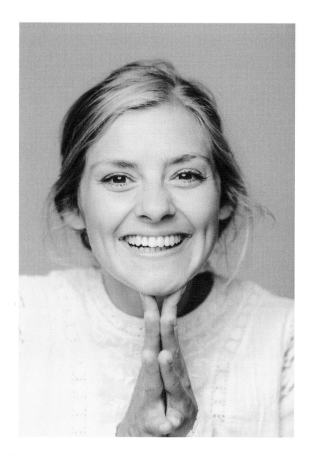

Hyggelig to meet you.

And welcome to *Hygge*. Even though this word might be new to you, I am sure you already know it from your own life. In a nutshell, it is a Danish word for finding happiness in *the little things in life.*

Hygge is said to be closely related to the Danish national character. But in its essence it is not Danish, it is universal. *Hygge* is for everyone – whoever you are, wherever you are.

My name is Marie Tourell Søderberg. I live in Copenhagen and work as an actress. As with most people these days, I sometimes feel caught up in my work. A rehearsal at the theatre is followed by a casting for a TV series, that is replaced by a session in the studio dubbing for a new Disney film – and I forget to take time to let it all go and let myself just *be*.

At these times it is crucial for me to have *hygge*. *Hygge* time with family and friends, *hygge* moments with myself and a *hyggelig* home.

Hygge has many shapes and forms – it looks different depending on who you ask. Over the course of the book you will meet a lot of Danes who explain how they *hygge* and what *hygge* is to them. You will also find inspiration on how to create a great basis for *hygge* to evolve in your everyday life.

For many Danes *hygge* is something you strive for. It's like a compass, steering us towards small moments that money cannot buy you, finding the magic in the ordinary.

Marie

To me, *hygge* is:

- *Meeting my sister for a walk in the park, chatting, laughing and clowning around, as if we were children again*
- *Listening to the rain on the roof with a cup of tea and my boyfriend next to me*
- *Drinking wine in my mum's garden*
- *Enjoying a cup of coffee with good friends, that becomes a dinner, that becomes a late-night drink, because no one wants the evening to end*

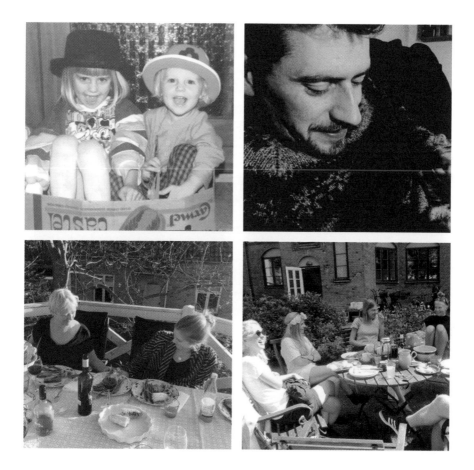

HOW TO

SPEAK *HYGGE*

When people from other countries talk about the Danish language they often say it is hard to learn. The grammar is very tricky and the pronunciation even trickier. Luckily, you don't have to learn Danish in order to 'speak *hygge*'.

66 I speak Spanish with my boyfriend, but we always use the term *hygge*-out when we have plans to do something *hyggelig*. Or *vamos* a *hygge*-out. I find it difficult now not to use the term when I speak with non-Danish people. I use 'cosy' to refer to all this, but I know it doesn't convey the full message of *hyggelig*. It's not that the concept of *hygge* doesn't exist in other cultures, but having a word for it makes you aware of it. All of a sudden you start to become aware of the many *hyggelig* parts of your everyday life.99

Júlia Reig from Catalonia,
living with her boyfriend in Copenhagen

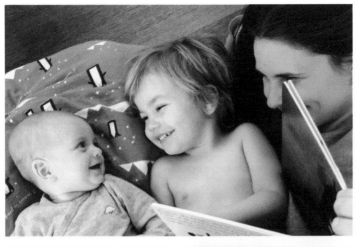

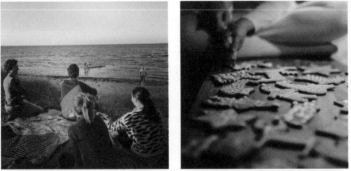

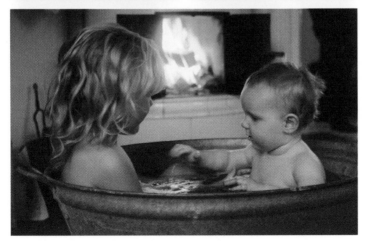

Useful *Hygge* expressions

The Danish word *hygge* is a verb, an adjective and a noun: we are *hygg*-ing (verb); the house is *hyggelig* (adjective); it is time for *hygge* (noun).

Hygger – Present tense of the verb 'to *hygge*', i.e. we are *hygg*-ing. Used to talk about doing a *hyggelig* activity or having a moment of *hygge*, e.g. 'What are you doing?' 'We are *hygg*-ing.'

Hyggliere/hyggeligste – More/most *hyggelig*. 'That is the *hyggeligste* place I've ever seen.'

Hygge om – *Hygge* around or make *hygge* for someone, e.g. serving them tea or snacks, making them comfortable, wrapping them in blankets or chit-chatting with them.

Hygge sig – To have a *hyggelig* time.

Hygge sig med – *Hygg*-ing oneself with something or having a *hyggelig* time doing something. Used to describe someone with a hobby, e.g. 'He is *hygg*-ing himself with playing the guitar'; 'We are *hygg*-ing with this do-it-yourself project.'

Kan du hygge dig/hyg dig – A popular Danish greeting or informal way of saying goodbye (literally 'Can you *hygge* yourself'/'*Hyg* yourself').

There are also many compound words formed with *hygge*, for example family-*hygge*, *hygge*-beer and *hygge*-snack. At the back of the book you will find a dictionary with lots more *hygge* compound words.

❝ *Hygge* is a state of being you experience if you are at peace with yourself, your spouse, the tax authorities and your inner organs.❞

Tove Ditlevsen, Danish writer and poet

Danes would be lost without the word *hygge*. They tell each other how much they are looking forward to *hygge* together, they point out how *hyggelig* a situation is while they are *hygging*, and afterwards they like to talk about what a great *hygge* time they have had together.

The word originates from the proto-language Old Norse – *hyggja* means thinking and feeling satisfied and is related to finding shelter, rest and safety, and regaining energy and courage.

The impact of the words we use

66 Within the newer branch of psychology, called narrative therapy, we talk about our identity being created by the stories we tell about ourselves and each other. Therefore, the language and the words we use and have available to us are crucial to who we are and how we understand ourselves.

In the original Inuit culture in Greenland, there are over twenty different words for snow. That not only makes it possible for Inuits to share the experiences of the various types of snow, it also sharpens their attention to nuances in the weather and helps to broaden their experience of nature's richness and diversity.

That's what it's like with *hygge*. The better able we are to talk about *hygge* and all its nuances and forms, the better able we are to realize it, create it and share it.

The word is not just a passive signifier, but a performative statement that does something for us and sets the stage in certain ways. When we call an experience '*hyggelig*', we associate – perhaps unconsciously – a range of values with this experience. In that way, *hygge* claims its place in the stories and narratives about who we are and what we value.99

Torkild Fogh Vindelev,
psychologist

[hYg:ə]

If you want to start including *hygge* in your own daily vocabulary, it might be good to be able to pronounce it properly.

Many people mistakenly think that *hygge* is pronounced something like *hooga* when they see the word for the first time. But if you want to sound like a native, here is a little guide* to how you do it. Let's take it step by step.

The last part of the word is pretty straightforward, so let's try that first. The 'gge' in *hygge* is the same 'gir' sound as in 'girl'. That's pretty easy.

Then the more troubling part will be the 'y' in *hygge*. Try to think of the 'y' as the 'ou' sound in 'you'. The vowel sound in 'you' is a diphthong (a vowel sound containing two different sounds) – 'y-ou'. Look at your mouth in the mirror and see it changing shape as you make the sound. The first part makes the lips do nearly nothing; the second part makes them round a bit. The 'y' sound in *hygge* is not a diphthong, it is a single vowel sound, so we must try to edit out the last part, the 'ou' sound that makes your mouth go round. What do we have left? The 'y' sound we need to pronounce *hygge* properly. Add an 'h' sound at the beginning and you've got it – *hygge*.

WHERE DOES *HYGGE*

COME FROM?

A Short Look into the Culture and History of *Hygge*

Different nations have different key values that underpin the way they understand and characterize themselves. The Americans are fond of individual freedom, the French have their *gloire* and the Germans favour order and precision. Among the people of Denmark, *hygge* would certainly be one of the key values.

The phenomenon has evolved in a melting pot consisting of the Danish climate, a history of being small, a home-orientated culture, the welfare state and equality, according to Professor Jeppe Trolle Linnet, who has studied the nature of *hygge*.

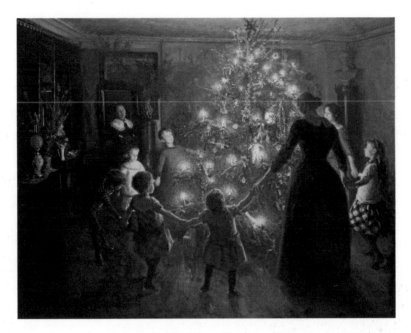

Viggo Johansen, Merry Christmas, 1891

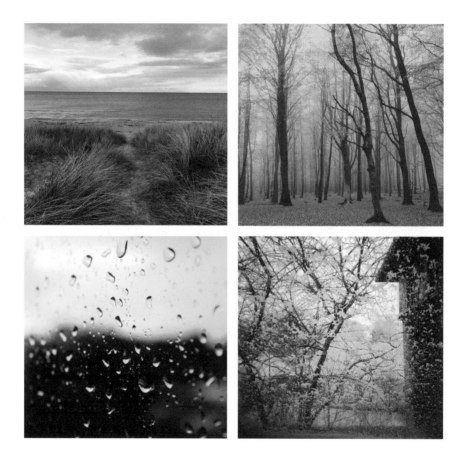

The Nordic climate features great contrasts between warmth and cold, light and darkness. We have long, light summer nights, but in winter the light hours fade away, and during the darkest time of the year a day has only between seven and eight hours of daylight. 'Grey and cloudy' is a frequent message from the Danish meteorologists when they forecast the next day's weather on TV. It rains approximately 171 days a year while the average temperature is around 17 degrees in summer and just above freezing point in winter. The slightly depressing weather forecasts have given Danes the urge to seek for warmth and comfort, which we mostly find at home, where we create room for companionship with our family and closer relations. As Jeppe Trolle Linnet, professor of *hygge*, explains:

66 Our unsettled climate has been a contributing factor as to why the Nordic cultures to some extent romanticize the home as a 'safe haven' where families get together and gather new strength to once again face the outside world. Home is the physical part of *hygge*, what the family is for the social part: the *hygge* in its proto form. When we seek *hygge* outside of our homes, it is mostly in places that have home-like features: limited view from the outside and in, dimmed lighting and comfortable furnishing. 99

Hygge is also rooted in the Danish history of being reduced in size. Once, areas of Sweden, Germany and Norway – even occasionally parts of Britain – were Danish, but gradually we lost it all, piece by piece. Losing Norway in 1814 meant losing the epic mountains, and Denmark became as flat as a pancake, while an escalating conflict between a belligerent Prussian Bismarck and a naive Danish government with megalomania resulted in a loss of one-third of the population and most of our national pride in 1864.

What could we do then? The only solution seemed to be to get the most out of the small and flat country that was left and our national saying became: 'What is lost on the outside shall be won on the inside,' a quote from the Danish poet H. P. Holst, meaning: Let's cultivate our land and enlighten ourselves.

66 We fostered a strong sense of community by forming groups and associations for people with shared interests or aims and we founded a new kind of school that was meant to enlighten the broader part of the population. These schools are known as Danish Folk High Schools.99

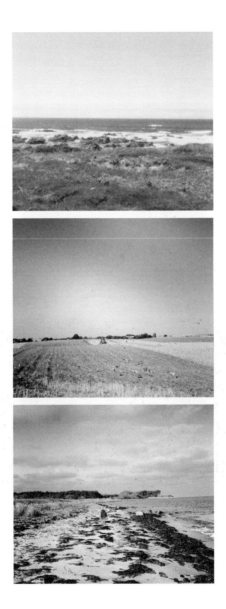

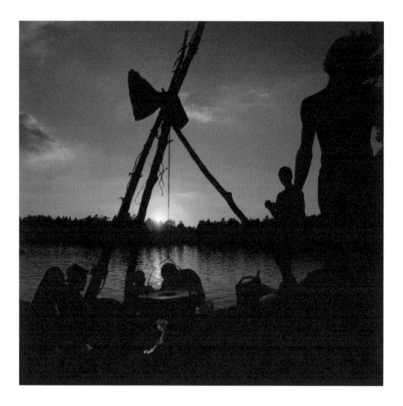

In the nineteenth century the first thoughts about the values, that later became the foundation of a modern welfare society, began to spring up:

66 In wealth, we have come far, when few have too much and fewer too little.99

N. F. S. Grundtvig (1783–1872),
pastor, poet, philosopher, historian, teacher and politician

This quote is said to have been the credo behind the Danish welfare policy for more than a hundred years. Denmark is well known for its welfare system and is considered to be one of the most egalitarian societies in the world, since the redistribution of resources evens up the gap between rich and poor. The provision of free education, healthcare and unemployment benefits gives Danes a feeling of economic security. When the basic needs are met, there is more room for one to explore the social, creative and personal elements of one's life – and it is easier for *hygge* to thrive.

66 The economic equalizing and a morality that emphasizes the subjective happiness of the individual, gives people the possibility, space and freedom to take a *hygge*-break and strive a little less. We don't have to struggle all the time.99

The characteristics of *hygge* as being peaceful, intimate, introvert and equalizing correspond with the self-image we have as a nation: a small and peaceful country that does not harm anyone and where everyone is equal, Jeppe Trolle Linnet concludes:

    " *Hygge* is universal and accessible for everyone. It is an integral part of being human and not exclusively Danish. But there are elements within *hygge* that correspond particularly well with the Scandinavian welfare state and with the Danish national self-awareness of being a small country."

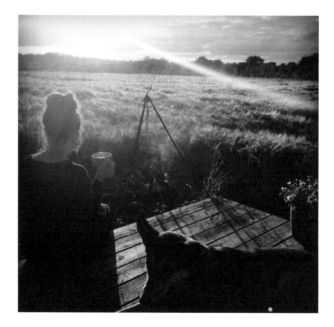

66 On a film set, it actually becomes very clear what it is we carry with us. An equal structure, first and foremost. I see this as something very Danish. We do not sit and hide inside our trailers or walk around and think we're special because we're actors. We are used to seeing ourselves as part of a team and we walk around chatting with everyone. Community lies very deep within us. Much deeper than most people realize, I think. 99

Danish actor Lars Mikkelsen, known from the TV series *House of Cards* and *The Killing*, in an interview in *Ud og Se* magazine

TOGETHERNESS

Many of the researchers who have dug into why Denmark is one of the happiest countries in the world have pointed at *hygge* as a contributing factor.

Personally, this is what makes me happy:

- Spending time with my boyfriend, family and good friends
- Working on inspiring and immersive projects
- Eating fantastic food in good company
- Enjoying a good book or small handiwork project
- Taking dancing classes
- Meditating
- Laughing
- Travelling with people I love

When I look at my list, togetherness seems to be central. In the time spent with family and friends, *hygge* plays a major part. I meet my friends and family with the express purpose of *hygg*-ing and I feel that sharing a sincere moment of *hygge* brings us even closer to each other.

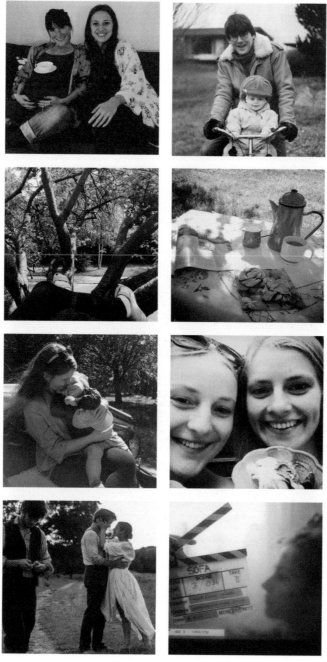

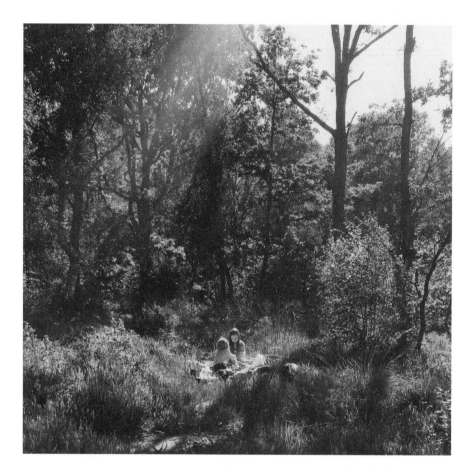

66 It is through *hygge* that we find and build really strong relationships with other people. There is an effortlessness in *hygge*, which means that we can be together with friends and family without having any plans besides relaxing and enjoying a good time together. We dare to be who we are in each other's company, and this affirms us that we have stable relationships in our lives, meaning we will never stand alone. This is a social security of great value, and one of the most important sources of our happiness.

In *hygge* we also find a sincerity and comfort that means that we dare to express ourselves when we disagree. And when we, in a respectful and relaxed way, dare to discuss the bigger questions in life, we get the opportunity to see ourselves and the life we lead with a new perspective, becoming more aware of what makes us happy. At the same time this new perspective opens our eyes to what we are able to change in order to improve our wellbeing.

It is not in *hygge* that we find ecstatic, and often momentary, happiness, but we experience a kind of everyday happiness. *Hygge* contributes to a general contentedness in the long run. 99

Christian Bjørnskov, Professor at Aarhus University
and author of *Lykke* (Happiness)

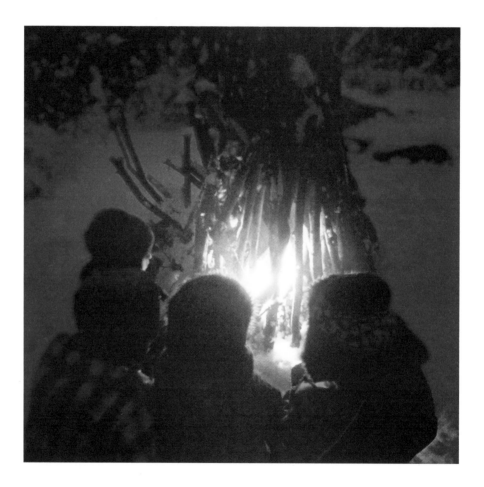

Hygg-ing Together

Having strong relationships is vital for our health and happiness, and *hygge* definitely helps us to do this by focusing our mind on time spent with loved ones. When we feel safe and comfortable with other people, the *hygge* becomes relaxed and authentic. Some people are exceptional at *hygg*-ing around other people and making them feel at ease. Meet twenty-eight-year-old Marendine Ladegaard and ninety-two-year-old Anna Elizabeth Gonge . . .

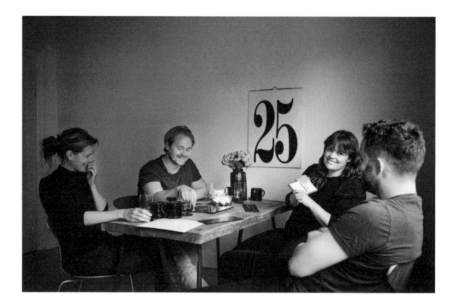

— I want my guests to feel at home

Marendine Ladegaard enjoys *hygg*-ing around her guests when they visit her at home. And she's good at it. Her circle of friends agree unanimously that she manages to create an informal atmosphere, where even though you're a guest, you feel at home, but at the same time you feel pampered. According to Marendine, it's about being a sincere and attentive host.

❝ Most importantly I want my guests to feel at home. I take it as a great compliment, for example, if they go into the kitchen, look in my cupboards and take what they need. It may be stepping over the line for some, but for me it's a sign that my guests feel comfortable.

When guests step inside, I try to sense where they are mentally and what they need. It is quite simple. If I can feel that they are tired after a long day at work, I'll ask if we should just curl up on the sofa and watch a TV show. If they come in from the cold, I'll offer them a blanket and a pair of home-knitted socks. I also often ask my guests if they would like to choose a cup, if we are to have something warm to drink. Then they may end up having a favourite cup here, and that helps them feel at home, I believe.

Sometimes guests can be in doubt about what to do with themselves when they come into someone's home, but if I say, 'Here's a glass of red wine, now sit down on the sofa,' then there's no worry, and it's easier for me to *hygge* around them.

Having energy for my guests is a main priority. Therefore, I lower my expectations for what I can manage to prepare for them, if I can see that I am short on time. I'd rather change the menu from a huge dinner to cheese and wine or sandwiches.

I'd also much rather invite friends and family home than meet them at a café in town. At home it's easier for me to set the framework of togetherness and, therefore, it is easier to create a relaxed, *hyggelig* and informal atmosphere. I throw my legs up on the sofa to indirectly show my guests that they are welcome to do the same, and I will tell my guests about a mistake I made at work, or that I am going to do a kayak test tomorrow, and I'm really nervous about it because I failed it the first time. It's about daring to share something about yourself and show that you're not infallible.

My guests need to have an unspoken knowledge that if they drop a cup and it breaks, then it'll be something we laugh at, not something we cry over.❞

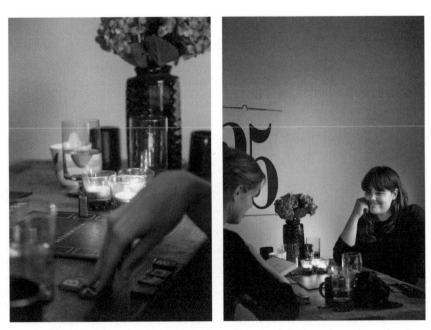

'I find that my guests and I achieve a familiarity and closeness much quicker at home than at a café. When I invite people home, I invest myself in them,' says Marendine Ladegaard (right photo)

– I'm a bit of a people person

Anna Elisabeth Gonge is a Visiting Friend for many of the
elderly people in her local area who are having a hard time,
either because of illness or because old age has taken hold.
While she is well and both health and mind are in top form,
she feels she might as well pass some of the care that she has
received during her life on to others.

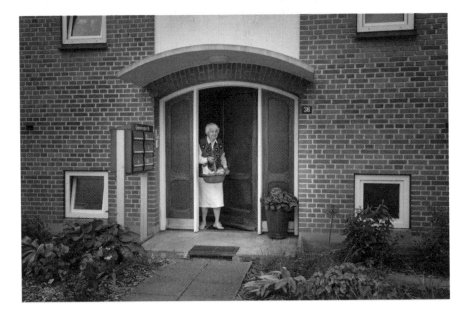

❝ I bring rolls and coffee with me when I go visiting, and I almost always start by asking how they feel. It is essential that the visit is on their terms, and it is important to listen. If they spend a large part of the day alone, they often have a lot to say. We talk about their health and how their family is doing and what the grandchildren are up to. Sometimes we sing together – songs they remember from their youth or evening songs. If they are in pain, we sometimes say a prayer for them. On the whole, it is about being present. When I feel that they are getting tired, I go home.

Sometimes I bring cake, and then it's best if it's apple cake, because everyone can chew that. We don't have so many teeth left – though the ones I have are my own, and they're quite secure! The coffee is the most important thing though, because then it doesn't matter if the conversation stops. Then we take just a sip of coffee and enjoy the silence for a moment.

I am a Visiting Friend because I am grateful for everything I've got over the years, so I think it's nice to give something back. And then I'm terribly fond of coffee and a bit of a people person.

To *hygge* yourself and feel good with others, that's life. It helps you retain a sharp mind. I've lost two daughters and my husband to a hereditary disease, and you need time to deal with that. But there comes a point when sorrow can't be allowed to fill your days and, instead, you have to be happy for all the good times you had together. I think that with a sharp mind and a little *hygge* every day, you can live a happy life in spite of what it throws at you.**"**

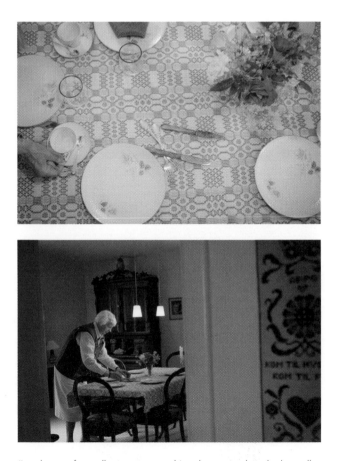

'I make sixty-four rolls at a time, and I make more when the last roll has been eaten. That way I always have something to share when I go visiting, and something to offer guests who come by. Sometimes I'll hang a bag of rolls on my neighbour's door handle, if I can see that he is home,' says Anna Elisabeth Gonge.

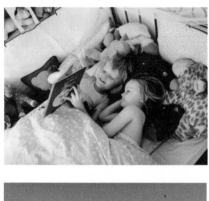

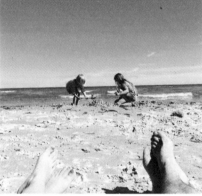

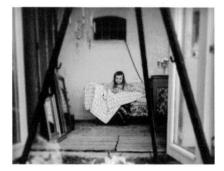

Why Children are Brilliant at *Hygging*

66 We had taken six months off from work, bought an auto camper and headed out in the world to be together as a family. The children were three and four years old at the time. After camping down through Europe and Morocco, we came to Greece, where we settled on the beach for a while. One day we saw a tortoise on its way down to the water. The children followed the tortoise's journey hour by hour; curiously observing its breaks, how it sought the shadow and routes through the sand.

When the tortoise finally reached the water, it dipped its feet, paddled a little, and chose to go back.

Astounded, and with sand on their knees, the children reflected on the tortoise's decision, while they – happily wondering – continued to follow the footprints of the tortoise back to where it came from. A whole day went by this way, and we were thrilled to have time to let them just be.99

Ole Viby, Sønder Nærå, Funen

Children are in many ways natural *hygge* experts. They experience the world with inspiring enthusiasm and wonder and they manage to create *hygge*: seeking out hidey-holes and places to play. They inspire us to just be in the here and now. It is hard to predict anything when we are with children.

❝ *Hygge* is when I read bedtime stories to my children. That is a ritual in our family – it is something we do every evening and that has always been a *hyggelig* moment, where we are drawn into fairy-tale universes together or gain knowledge about all kinds of things; from how the bees make honey to miscellaneous facts about Star Wars figures. It is a moment with presence, when we sit closely together. This closeness is for me the quintessence of *hygge.*❞

Tilde Vengsgaard,
teacher and mother of three, Randers

Danish Children are Brought Up with *Hygge*

Danish children learn the value of being part of a community and gain trust in themselves and others in their *hygge*-hours with Mum and Dad, says psychologist and author of *The Danish Way of Parenting*, Iben Sandahl.

What function does hygge *have in Danish families?*

66 For many families *hygge* is the 'glue' that holds the family together. It is in the *hygge* that we feel each other's presence, feel connected, and it is where each individual family member sees themselves again. Today, the everyday lives of Danish children are so packed with activities that planned *hygge*-time is mostly for the weekends. But some manage to integrate *hygge* during the week by putting small moments of it into the rhythm and routines already in place. It may be singing a song on the way home from kindergarten or telling jokes over dinner and laughing together. 99

Are Danish children brought up to hygge *themselves?*

❝ To a great extent. Children mirror and soak up everything from the moment they are born. They copy their everyday behaviour from Mum and Dad, kindergarten, friends and the people and the modern influences they interact with. A newborn is dependent on body and eye contact, care, attention and essential cognitive stimulation – this need and this human contact can be equated with the satisfaction and joy that results from *hyggelig* contexts; we feel stimulated, seen, heard and recognized. In most cases, *hygge* for kids is centred around the home – where they feel safe and secure, but have free space.❞

What does it mean to children that hygge *is included in their upbringing?*

66 It means that they know the significance of community and being present. If they have experienced their parents' presence often during their childhood, they know what it feels like to feel confirmed in a purely existential way – I have been seen, heard and met. They feel fundamentally safe, and if you feel safe as a human being, it is easier to deal with the external demands and expectations of everyday life. At the same time, *hygge* being part of a child's upbringing means that when children interact with other people, they find it easier to tune in to when relationships feel trustworthy and safe. This 'we-culture' is created in *hygge*; 'we find safety in each other' and 'we share this experience' is what we build our society on – a community-orientated society. 99

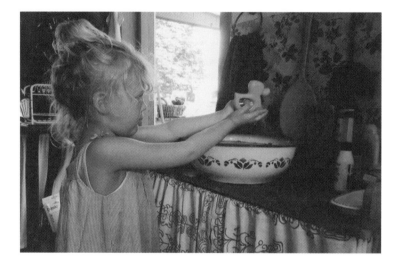

Making *Hygge* a Priority

The demands of everyday life challenge daily *hyggelig* moments in the family, but it is possible to plan for more time together, according to psychologist Heidi Schøitz:

66 Involve your children in practical tasks – assign chores to each of them. Let them help prepare food and try to eat together as often as possible. We often end up doing everything ourselves based on the idea that 'it'll be faster, and then we can *hygge* afterwards', but it can be very *hyggelig* to do practical things together. When we involve our children in everyday chores, we are also teaching them to take care of themselves. This strengthens the children's self-confidence, self-esteem and independence.

Look at your time-budget too – what are you actually spending your time on? Electronic paraphernalia are often significant time-wasters, so try to put the phones away and turn off computers, TVs and iPads when the family is gathered around an activity or during dinner. Lower your ambitions too, make a meal plan and do a food shop once a week. 99

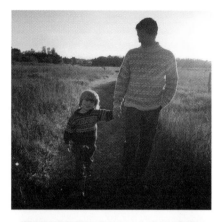

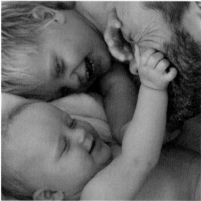

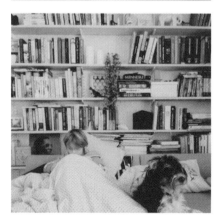

In my nephew's kindergarten, this sign was put up just before the Easter holidays:

> ❝ Don't forget to have some potter-time. It is important for the children to have time to potter around in slippers without all those well-meaning plans of going to the zoo, the cinema or all kinds of other doings. ❞

'Pottering' means walking around with little effort or purpose, and it is about winding down and seeing that the *hygge* simply can hide within a pair of slippers.

The Unexpected and Spontaneous *Hygge*

Hygge can be stimulated, facilitated and prioritized but it can also evolve when we least expect it. Something is cancelled, the metro stops, there is no electricity – we have to wait, and waiting time can become a chance to spend time together.

My boyfriend and his parents and three sisters once got caught in a snowstorm when he was a child. And what should have been a nice two-hour evening drive home from dinner with relatives ended up being an eight-hour trip in their old Ford car because of an almost blocked motorway and lines of slowly moving cars as far as the eye could see. It could have been a terrible, long and exhausting journey home, but instead he remembers it as something extremely *hyggelig*: the snow, the big family cramped together in the car, playing games and talking through it all – and the shared memory it has become.

When *Hygge* Disappears

66 You can't just say 'now we *hygge*', and then expect *hygge* to show up. Exactly like you can't say 'now I want to fall in love'.99

Iben Sandberg, psychologist,
author of *The Danish Way of Parenting*

You can try to coax *hygge*, but you cannot force it. It will not work if we demand 'I have ten minutes to spare, let's *hygge*'! It has its own ways, and it comes and goes with the good spirit and atmosphere. A planned *hygge*-evening which had so much *hygge* potential can end up less *hyggelig* than intended if our expectations get too high and our plans too meticulous.

66 To me, *hygge* is a moment of letting go – a moment without limitations of time, duties, stress or distractions. A moment of love, warmth and time to gather round the small things: a card game, a book or a bath. When I look at my girls sharing a laugh or when I cuddle up in the corner of the couch with them. *Hygge* is that extra time I give myself to fully enjoy a special moment but at the same time something that magically happens every single day if I simply open my eyes.99

Nanna Mosegaard,
mother of two, Nørrebro, Copenhagen

Hygge Then and Now

Does age mean something to our understanding of what *hygge* is and is there a difference between *hygge* today compared to sixty years ago? Twenty-seven-year-old Lea Sommer was a child in the 1990s and associates *hygge* with listening to podcasts and a barbeque on weekend evenings, while for her ninety-year-old grandmother, Grete, *hygge* is enjoying the crossword and a little schnapps. They meet each other on the couch where *hygge* materializes, relaxing in each other's company.

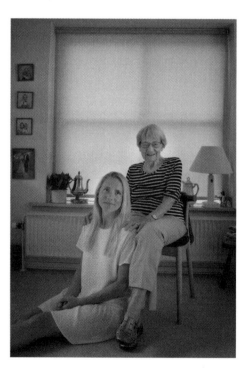

Lea:

Hygge is very much a state for me. When I am *hygg*-ing, I am present. I let go of the past and the future and I am content. I don't need anything other than what there is.

Grete:

You've hit the nail on the head there. For me, *hygge* can happen even if I'm alone. For example, when I sit with the Sunday paper and do the crossword. Everything is peaceful, I am present. But sometimes it is difficult to find the peace crucial for having a *hyggelig* time, isn't that right?

Lea:

Definitely, and when I can't find peace, it's because my mind is racing. I'm worrying about something that has happened or will happen. Sometimes you can do something to actively create the peace that must be present for *hygge* to occur. If I'm alone and would like to *hygge*, I can take a long bath, cut my fruit a little fancy, light some candles and put on some music that reminds me of other *hyggelig* moments. Other times, I can feel a peace arising in me, and then *hygge* comes of its own accord.

Grete:

I am always more satisfied with myself on those days when I manage to do all those things I had planned to get done, and a feeling of *hygge* arises from that. 'Now it's all right to sit and *hygge* in the evening. It's well deserved now,' I say to myself.

Lea:

When do you typically seek a *hygge* moment for yourself?

Grete:

Saturday evening. I never eat hot food then. Instead, I butter some sandwiches and make a nice little salad. And then I pour a single schnapps and half a beer. It is a Saturday tradition from the time your grandfather, Hans was alive. We had a little conversation, which we often repeated Saturday after Saturday. Hans would ask if we had any cod livers for dinner. 'Yes, indeed we do,' I always replied. We nearly always had some in the fridge. 'Shall we have some of them?' he'd ask. 'Let's have them with toasted bread and lemon. Will we have some schnapps too?' I'd ask. 'Yes, let's have two,' he'd reply, and that was how we planned dinner on a Saturday.

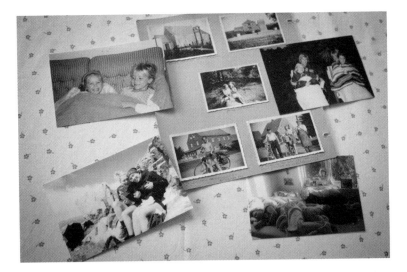

Lea:

Do you think about Grandad in your *hygge* moments on
Saturdays?

Grete:

Yes. I think of all the good years we had together. They are a
part of my *hygge*. Saturday dinner is a longstanding tradition
in our family. We introduced cold food on Saturday evenings
when the children were small. It was so nice to have one day
a week where I didn't have to think about planning a hot dinner.

Lea:

Yeah, and Dad took that tradition from his childhood and carried
it on at home with us. We often ate at eight o'clock on Saturdays
– rye bread and cold meats from the fridge. And we often sat
on the couch rather than around the dinner table. It was a real
hygge-moment. As a child it meant a lot to me to feel that my
parents relaxed so much on Saturday nights. It generated in
me a feeling of *hygge* and that was much more important than
having pizza, burgers or something more exotic. It was probably
also what made Saturdays so special rather than weekday
evenings.

Grete:

When I was a kid in the 1930s, I remember weekday evenings
in my childhood home being very *hyggelig*. Father would sit at
his desk, going through his papers or reading the newspaper,
while Mother sat knitting or doing other needlework. I clearly
remember the cat lying behind Mother's back as she sat working.

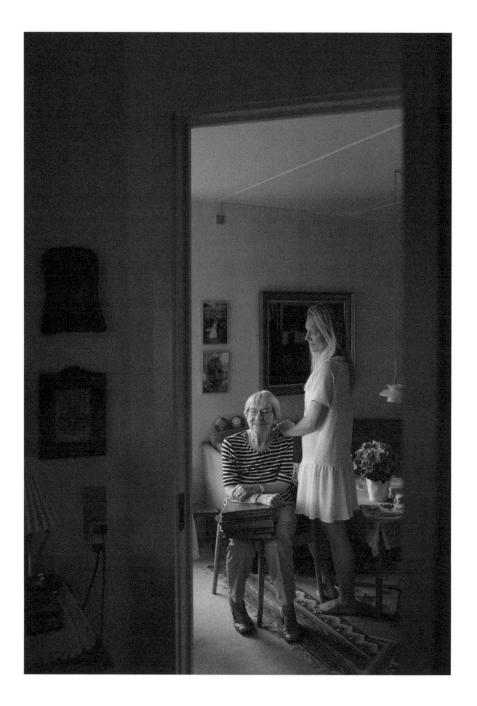

I often sat drawing or doing homework. Sometimes Father sat and drew with me. And at nine o'clock we had coffee. There were also nights where one of us would suggest a game of cards, and so we would play cards. We were never bored. Those *hyggelig* moments mean a lot to me. I felt safe.

Would you say that you are in harmony with yourself when you're *hygging*?

Lea:

Yes, having *hygge* in my life helps me to create harmony. I think that my life would be quite unhealthy if I wasn't good at *hygging* myself. It's in the *hygge* that I put life on pause and remember to enjoy the little things.

Grete:

When we are together the two of us, we are good at *hygging* ourselves. Isn't that right?

Lea:

Yeah, if it's an evening, we often end up on the couch, when I lay my head in your lap. And, at that moment, we don't focus on anything else.

Grete:

That's *hygge*.

Lea:

Yeah, that's *hygge*.

Going Out

A female commander-in-chief in the Danish Security and
Intelligence Service, a man who dresses as a woman, old
friends and friends who haven't yet decided whether they
want to be more than friends; everyone meets in the pub.
The pub is an all-embracing cave, where the *hygge* settles in
with the crackling of a candle, the regular waiter's nod of
recognition and the lowering of barriers.

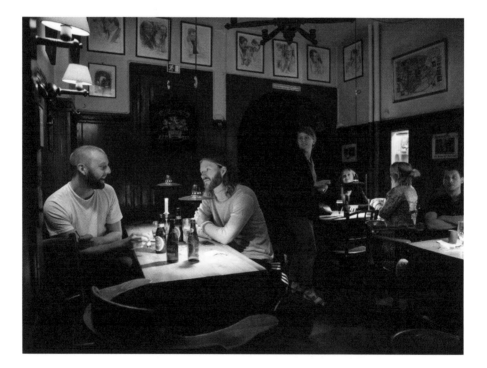

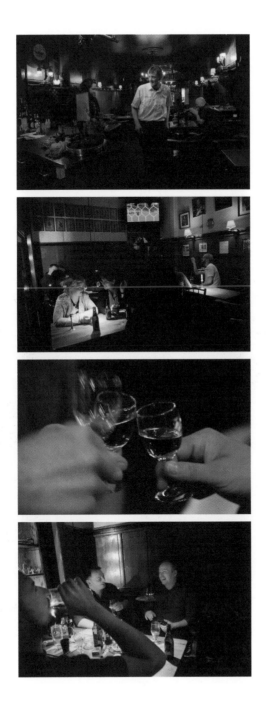

Every evening at 6 o'clock 150 to 200 people meet to dine together in a disused church in Copenhagen. Sitting shoulder to shoulder are tired families with children, smiling grandparents, and neighbours who want to get to know each other but don't have space in their own apartments. It is the founder of the Tiger store chain, Lennart Lajboschitz, who bought the church in 2014 and turned it into a modern community centre, which, besides communal dining, also holds yoga classes, board game competitions and talks. 'This is an extension of your living room. Let the *hygge* begin,' says Morten, the chef, when he introduces the menu of the evening.

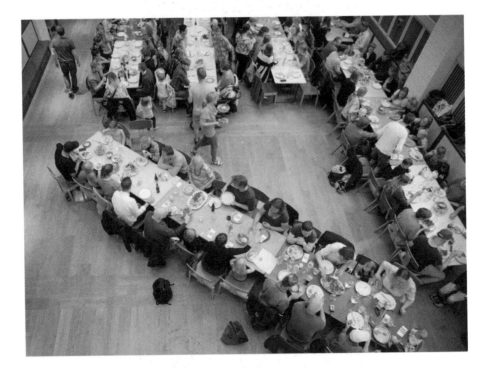

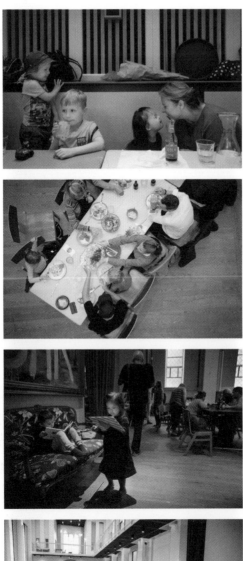
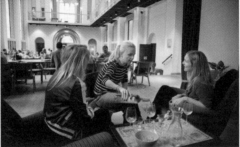

INVITING *HYGGE*

TO THE TABLE

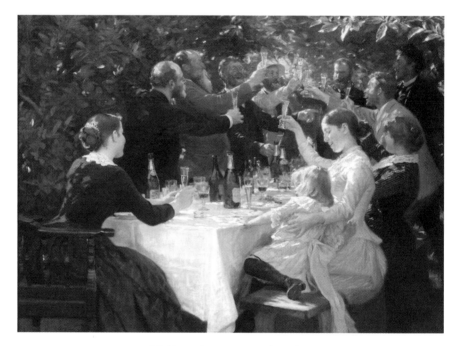

P.S. Krøyer, Hip, Hip, Hurrah!, 1888

Thousands of years ago, we were hunter-gatherers. After catching our food, we made a fire and prepared the meal – and enjoyed it together. The fire became the central place of warmth and light and the culture of togetherness in eating evolved.

Now our hunting for meat takes place in the refrigerator in the supermarket – but we still prefer the social aspects of enjoying the meal together. The feast has become fundamental to our social life.

Talking and evaluating the day around the table was the central part of everyday family life for me. Sometimes my mother, father, sister and I would sit there for a long time, eating and chatting about what had happened during the day. At other times, dinner was replaced by homework and cups of tea. The big dining table in our living room was our primary place of family togetherness.

Homemade Food

66 *Hygge* is cooking food with my boyfriend in our kitchen, while our daughter plays on the floor. Or making a picnic basket that we bring to our small boat to eat. *Hygge* is when I bake a cake or when my boyfriend makes a fantastic dish out of a seemingly empty fridge, when we have unexpected guests.99

Neel Rønholt, Copenhagen

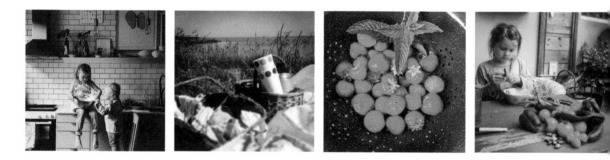

The personal element and wonderful smell of something homemade underlines that what you are about to eat is authentic and unique and far away from mass production.

Investing time and energy in a homemade dinner or a homebaked cake adds a feeling of *hygge* to a gathering around the table. The food itself doesn't have to be advanced or fancy. If it's down-to-earth, it adds to the *hygge* rather than distracting from it.

HYGGELIG RECIPES

AUNTY INA'S THICK PANCAKES

Ina Schack Vestergaard is sixty-one years old, married to Søren, and is a mother of three and grandmother of five. She lives on Ærø, a small island in southern Denmark with just 6,000 inhabitants. Ærø residents are known to be a proud, seafaring people and are famous for their hospitality and their thick pancakes. Family recipes for the small, oval treats are often passed from generation to generation, and opinions on how to make the best pancakes have been shared loudly for as long as Ina can remember. They must be neither too heavy, too greasy, too airy, too oval nor too round.

" There are as many opinions about how to make thick pancakes as there are about parenting and how to lacquer a ship. Therefore, it is only within the last ten years that I have dared to start making thick pancakes. Like many of Ærø's young inhabitants today, I thought it was terribly difficult, and I was worried that people would do a double-take at the thickness, shape and airiness of my pancakes. But it's actually quite easy to make Ærø pancakes. This recipe is my own, but it's based on inspiration from a local priest's family's recipe and Mother Issi's recipe. Mother Issi is the mother-in-law of my husband's brother. She was a colourful character, who always made her pancakes while wearing cotton knickers on her head to avoid getting fat in her hair. She even kept the knickers on her head when she got unexpected visitors. It didn't bother her in the slightest, and when she made pancakes, she made so many she could feed the entire town.

Thick pancakes are good for afternoon tea, evening tea and unexpected guests. The beauty of them is that I can make a lot of pancakes at once and freeze them. When I see people coming to the door, I just heat a few pancakes on the stove, and it's like they've been freshly made. That way I always have something to offer my guests. When my children and grandchildren dock with the ferry on Friday night, coming over for a weekend visit, I have a cup of tea and a pancake ready for them. For the annual accordion festival, I – and sixteen other of the island's ladies – make 1,600 thick pancakes for the festival's guests. They work for any occasion. "

Ina Schack Vestergaard

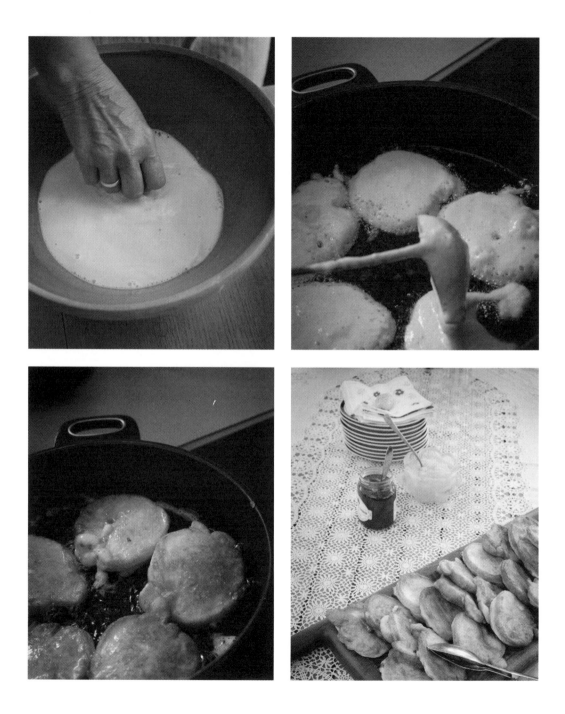

Makes approx. 35 pancakes

500ml milk

50g fresh yeast

8 to 10 eggs (*Tip from Else Grydehøj's grandmother:* never skimp on the eggs!)

500g flour

Pinch of salt

Pinch of sugar

Lard – plenty (or sunflower oil)

Warm the milk and stir in the yeast. The milk should be 'little-finger warm'.

Separate the egg yolks and egg whites. Add the flour, yolks, salt and sugar together and mix to a batter. Pour boiling water into a large dish and place the batter in a water bath (to raise the batter and get the most out of it – as is the frugal spirit of Ærø's residents).

Whisk the whites until stiff and then fold them into the batter while it is still in the water bath. Melt the lard or sunflower oil in a pot. Hold the wooden end of a match in the fat to see if it sizzles – if it does, it is hot enough. With the ladle pour some fat from the pot into the saucepan, filling it up so that it is just over 1cm deep. (Now hold your tongue – and put children and telephones on silent.)

Fill the ladle with batter and pour it into the pan to form five oval-shaped pancakes about 1 cm deep and 8 cm in diameter. The first pancake is turned over when the fifth is properly floating on the fat. It shouldn't be in the pan for too long. Whenever you start a new batch of pancakes, pour new fat into the pan. It is important that the fat has a depth of just above 1 cm all the time. The pancakes must not touch the bottom or float too high, they should just float easily. (This takes practice.)

The finished fried pancakes are immediately placed on newspaper, to absorb the excess fat.

Tip: Serve with gooseberry compote, jam or stewed apple/rhubarb.

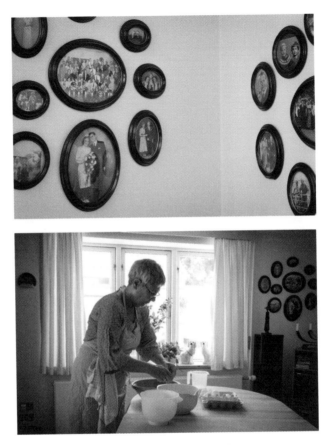

The two porcelain dogs in the background can be seen on windowsills around the island. The story goes that when the man of the house is home from sailing, the dogs face inwards, but when the man is out sailing, the dogs face outwards. Whether they are scouting for their masters or a sign that the woman's lover can come to visit is hard to know.

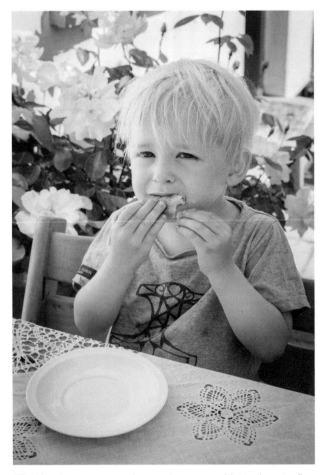

Alfred, Ina's youngest grandson, is three years old. He doesn't talk when he eats his pancakes and he can eat at least four in a row. Alfred has a trick for the jam, too – he licks the jam off first. That way he can spread more jam on his pancakes and have twice as much.

PALLE'S MORNING ROLLS

Palle is married to Edith and has been for over thirty years. Together they have four children, and for a large part of their lives they have worked together at a Danish boarding school in northern Jutland. When you know each other as well as Palle and Edith do, and have shared both life's sunny and dark sides, you know that it is important to continue to make each other happy in everyday life. Even if it's just by baking fresh rolls, Palle says.

66 Normally, I'm not a person who spends much time in the kitchen. I am far better at eating food than making it. But I like to bake bread, and I do it often. It's the only time I feel at home in the kitchen apart from when I'm doing the dishes or peeling potatoes.

When I bake rolls, I make the dough the evening before. It takes maybe twice as long as brushing your teeth, so it's not long. In the morning, I wake up a bit before the alarm goes off, typically around six a.m., and then I get up, put on my slippers and go into the kitchen. Edith likes to sleep a little longer, and while I get up as soon as the alarm goes off, she sleeps on soundly. We're different that way.

Within ten minutes I'll have shaped the rolls, sprinkled sesame seeds on them and put them in the oven. Then I make coffee and set the table as I listen to the radio. It has become a morning ritual that I like very much. Just like Dan Turell (a Danish poet), I like the everyday. Its repetition. In a life where everything moves quickly, and you have to be on top of everything, it's nice to have a morning routine. Something I just do without having to think about it too deeply. It gives me peace of mind to know exactly what I am going to do in the day's first hour and, actually, I believe it's healthy.

When the smell of freshly baked rolls has drifted to the bedroom, and I call, Edith wakes and comes down to the living room. It is wonderful to start the day together over a freshly baked roll. We both benefit from it. When you have lived together for thirty years, you know what the other person thinks before they say it aloud and vice versa. Sometimes you take each other for granted, and it's not always possible to think beyond yourself. But if you want to live together for many years, you have to continue to *see* each other. I know very well there is no art in baking rolls but, sometimes, I think of it as a way to show Edith that I am grateful to her and for what we have together, and that I like doing things that can make her happy. When we meet the day together in the morning before we head off in different directions, it affirms our cohesion. We are alive in relation to each other, and share something special together right there in that moment. 99

Palle Fogh, Aalborg

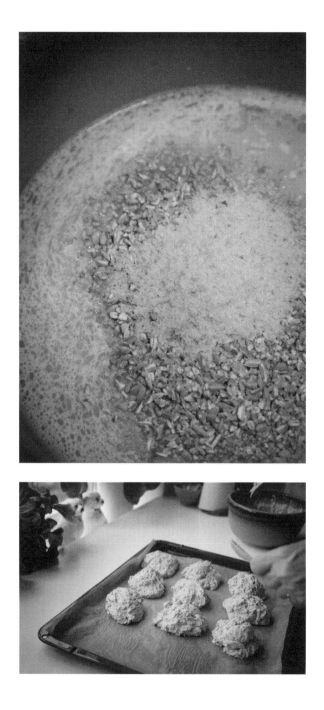

Makes 10 to 12 rolls

15g organic yeast

600ml cold water

1 tbsp sea salt

50g cracked wheat

50g cracked rye

400g wheat flour

150g spelt flour

50g coarse organic oatmeal

1 tbsp cold-pressed olive oil

Sesame seeds to sprinkle on top

The evening before, dissolve the yeast in the water. Add the salt, cracked wheat and cracked rye. Add all the flour and the oatmeal a little at a time. Mix the dough and refrigerate overnight.

In the morning, set the oven to 210° C. You don't have to knead the dough. Using two tablespoons, shape the dough into rolls. Brush them with oil and sprinkle them with sesame seeds, then bake for 22 minutes.

Serve warm to someone you care about. Enjoy them, for example, with butter and cheese, an optional piece of red pepper or a blob of jam on top.

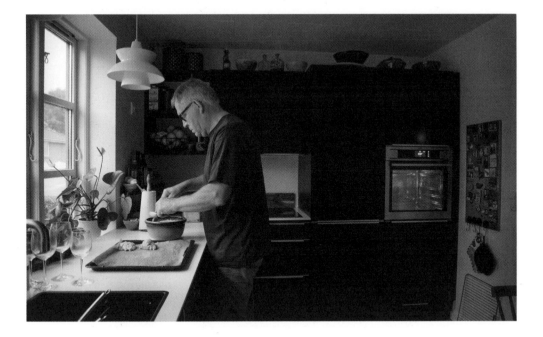

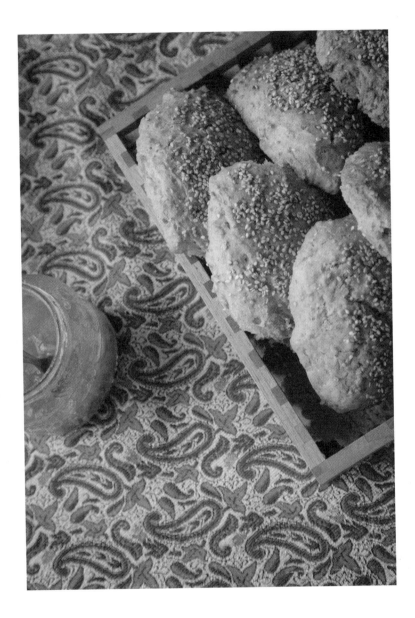

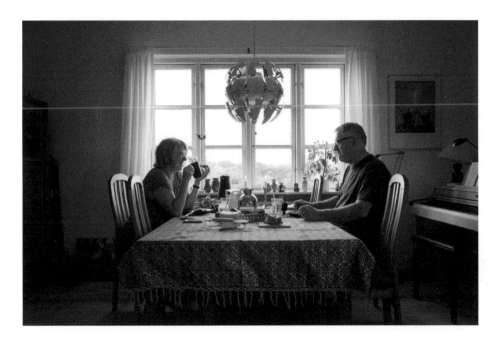

LOUISE'S POTATO SANDWICHES — WITH CRUNCH

66 When I was a child the whole family often gathered around potato sandwiches at lunchtime and we still eat them together when we go to my family's farm in Sweden during the holidays and at weekends. Potatoes, homemade rye bread, radishes, butter, mayonnaise and chives are all placed on the large kneading board – a wooden board that is found under the kitchen table in many Swedish farms. Then the kneading board is carried out. We always eat outside when we are in Sweden, even in rain and sleet. We sit together under the overhang from the little farm and we butter, build and eat our potato sandwiches. Very *hyggelig* to me.

Potato sandwiches are also a sure-fire summer classic when I invite my girlfriends home. They are a classic of traditional Danish *smørrebrød* – open sandwiches – and I value good ingredients that are not available throughout the year, but are especially delicious and fresh in certain seasons. In winter, we have to make do with the chalk-white, dull potatoes. But then suddenly they are here: the fledgling new potatoes. Along with the strawberries and rhubarb and everything else that blooms in early summer. I am one of those people who always buys an over-priced tray of the first new potatoes in May, because I just can't wait any longer.

I once heard a chef say that the fewer ingredients there are in a dish, the less you have to compromise on the quality of the raw materials. That's my starting point when it comes to potato sandwiches. Here, I allow myself to splurge a little extra on good rye bread from the bakery, and I like to make mayonnaise from the eggs of hens that have lived well.

Hygge has a curious nature. It often occurs when I combine something I have done many times before with a new place. For example, having a potato sandwich in one of my favourite places in Copenhagen – the gunboat sheds on Holmen, enjoying it with my legs dangling in the water and the sun warming my skin.**"**

Louise Kjeldsen, Copenhagen

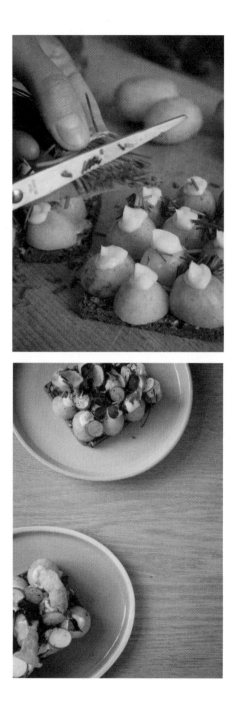

Serves 2

Rye bread (or another dark bread, preferably homemade)

Butter

New potatoes, cooked and cooled

Radishes

Chives or the top of a spring onion, chopped

Something crunchy: bacon or root vegetable crisps

Something to decorate, such as sorrel or pansies

For homemade mayonnaise

2 egg yolks (at room temperature)

Pinch of salt

A little lemon juice

A little mustard (optional)

About 120ml of neutral-tasting oil (grapeseed oil or sunflower oil)

Beat the first four mayonnaise ingredients with an electric mixer, then add the oil a little at a time while beating until the mixture has the right consistency.

Now, butter a piece of rye bread. Slice the potatoes and spread them out on the bread. Slice the radishes and put them on top of the potatoes. Top with the mayonnaise, and sprinkle chives or spring onion on top. Add the crunch and the decorations. And enjoy!

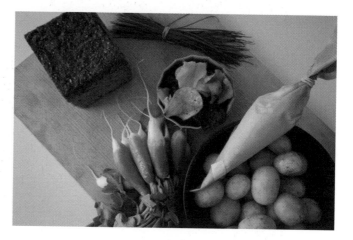

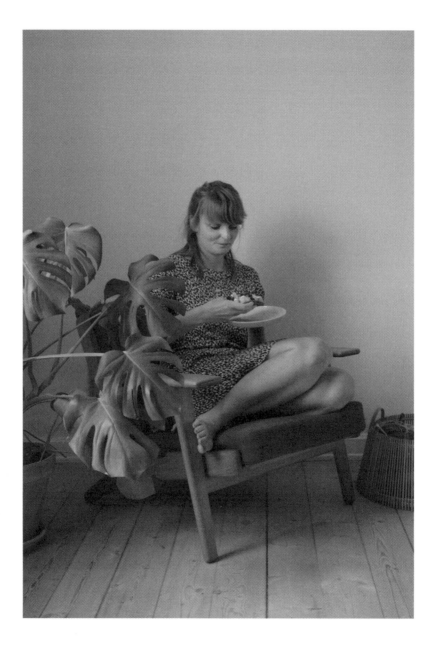

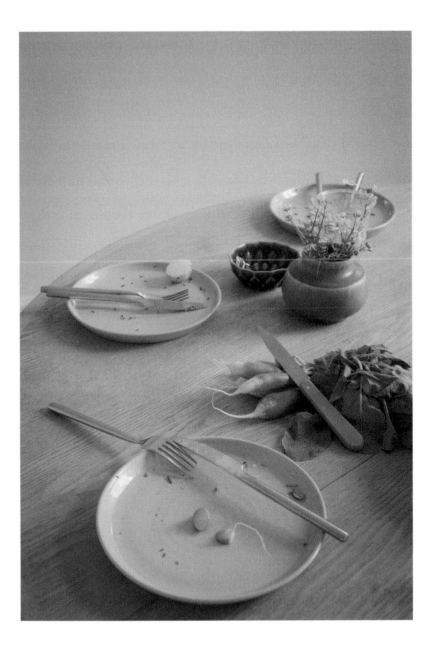

CAMILLA PLUM'S
RØDGRØD MED FLØDE
(SUMMER COMPÔTE)

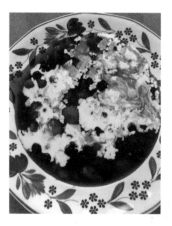

Rødgrød med fløde is a classic Danish dessert (and the name of the recipe is a classic tongue twister for foreigners).

This wonderful and famous compôte is basically a summer pudding without the bread: an intensely flavoured, lightly set compôte of mixed berries, with raspberries stirred in as it cools. Strewn with flaked almonds, then eaten with a thick blob of rich cream and a sprinkling of sugar to add crunch, this dessert is heaven on a long, light summer evening, and so special to the Nordic summer.

This is the recipe from the Danish chef Camilla Plum and her book *Cook Scandinavian*.

Serves 6–8

500g strawberries, hulled

500g black- or redcurrants and/or gooseberries

250–450g sugar

3 tbsp cornflour

500g raspberries (stir these in at the very end, when you remove the rest from the heat)

To serve:

cream

50g almonds, halved

Put the strawberries and the currants or gooseberries (don't bother topping or tailing these) into a wide non-corrosive pan. The amount of sugar needed varies enormously with the berries, but try 250g to start with. Add absolutely no water! Heat the pan gently and boil until the berries begin to release their juices. Lower the heat and let the fruit bubble away until the strawberries become *jammy* and the whole thing tastes like heaven.

Adjust the sugar: the compôte should be sweet, but still a little tart, and you must allow for a crunchy sprinkling of sugar when it's eaten. Dissolve the cornflour in a little juice from the berries and stir into the compôte, making sure that it is evenly distributed. Boil for another 5 minutes, remove from the heat, then stir in the raspberries and leave to cool.

When the compôte has cooled a little, pour it into a beautiful bowl and sprinkle generously with sugar to prevent a skin forming. When it is cold and set, decorate with the almonds. Eat cold with cream.

OATMEAL WITH CARAMEL SAUCE, APPLE AND ROASTED ALMONDS

Lasse Skjønning Andersen has revised the Danes' view on porridge by creating the artisan porridge boutique GRØD in Copenhagen. He has updated the plain porridge we know from our childhood and made it into a delicious treat.

66 Oatmeal with caramel sauce, apples and roasted almonds is the *hyggeligste* porridge for me because it has followed me since 2011, when I started GRØD. While other porridges have been changed along the way, that one has been there all along as my faithful companion. Customers like it, and I like it. It's a bit like a good friend you never grow tired of.99

Lasse Skjønning Andersen,
creator of GRØD in Copenhagen

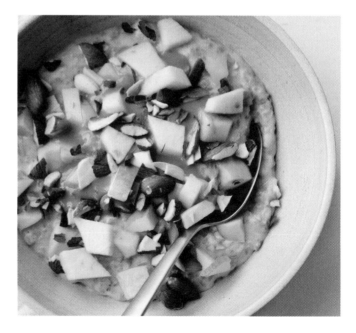

Serves 2

For the oatmeal

1½ cups rolled oats

1½ cups water

1½ cups milk

A bit of water

Salt

For the caramel sauce

(This will give you loads of caramel sauce, which you can keep in the fridge for 3–4 weeks.)

4 cans of condensed milk

¼ cup boiling water

For the topping

40g almonds

1 apple, chopped

Caramel Sauce

Put the cans of condensed milk into a saucepan and cover with water. Let the cans simmer for 4–5 hours. Top up the water if necessary so that the cans are always covered. After removing the cans carefully from the saucepan, run cold water over them until they have cooled down. Open the cans and blend the caramel liquid with a little boiling water until it has a creamy consistency.

Toppings

Roast the almonds in a pan over a medium heat until they're completely crisp and have a golden-brown colour. Chop the nuts before serving (you can roast more than you need and keep them in an airtight container).

Oatmeal

Bring the ingredients to the boil over a high heat. Then bring down to a medium heat and let it reduce to a nice consistency. (Takes about 7–8 minutes.) Season with salt.

To serve:

Serve the porridge in soup plates or bowls and top with a tablespoon of caramel sauce, chopped apples and roasted almonds.

SNOBRØD

Homemade, surrounded by nature, light, warmth and good
company – enjoying *snobrød* is a classic *hygge* moment and the
making of it stimulates all our senses: *smelling* the bonfire and
the chilly summer night, *seeing* the dancing flames, and *feeling*
the warmth on your face.

Snobrød – twisted rolls – is a way of making bread by twisting
some dough round a stick and baking it over the embers of a fire,
perhaps twisting it round a sausage for a more filling meal or just
eating it plain with jam.

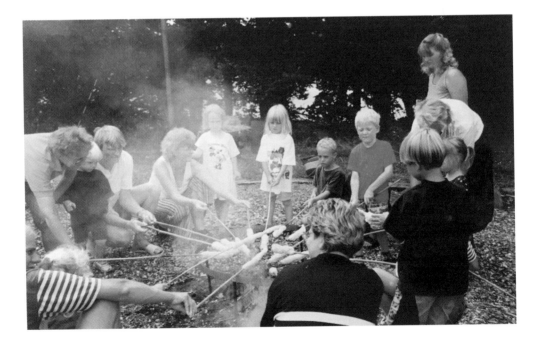

Makes 10 *snobrød/* twisted rolls

300ml full-fat milk or simply water

25g yeast

1 tsp salt

500g flour

A little bit of sugar and cardamom to sweeten

10 sharpened sticks with the ends stripped of bark

Gently heat the milk or water until it is lukewarm. Add the yeast and dissolve it. Add the salt and little by little add the flour, then a pinch of sugar and cardamom. Knead the dough then let it rest for 30 minutes. (You can strip the bark off the sticks and sharpen them while you are waiting for the bread to rise.)

Make 10 small sausage-shaped pieces out of the dough and twist each one round a stick. (If you go for the sausage version, wrap the dough around the sausage.) Leave the dough to rise for a further 20 minutes.

Bake the rolls over the fire until they are golden. Enjoy them as they are or with jam and butter.

Hygge Snacks

People from other countries notice that Danes often bring homemade cakes and buns to birthday celebrations in school, to work when we leave to go on holiday, or when we prepare for a moment of *hygge* after a piece of work.

For many years now, I have been known among my friends as the one who always brought her own snacks. I always had something sweet in my lunch box at school. Later on it became a snack in the handbag. To me, snacks equal *hygge*! But quite soon I discovered that I would be in trouble if I kept *hygg*-ing the way I did, snacking like that several times a day, whenever I had a *hygge*-moment.

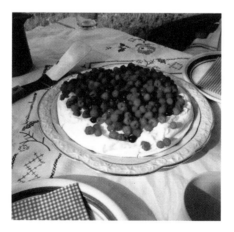

Hygge . . . and Health

Danes are the second highest sweet-eating nation in Europe and the reason is *hygge* – according to Heidi Boye, a consumer specialist and researcher, who has investigated how the phenomenon of *hygge* influences the Danes' relationship with food and sweets:

      66 When I say to my four-year-old son that we will really *hygge* ourselves tonight, he's not thinking of carrot sticks and broccoli florets. For the vast majority of Danes *hygge* is closely associated with drinking and eating, and it is often quite unhealthy treats that are set on the table. Treats are a ritual that communicates a transition from a hard-working weekday to well-earned leisure time. The busier we are – the more shopping lists there are to be written, bills to be paid and emails to be answered – the more we strive for *hygge*. *Hygge* is the antithesis of the rat race. We deserve a break from the demands of work and the advice of health experts and, therefore, we consume sweets in *hygge*'s name without that much of a guilty conscience. 99

SNICKERS

A couple of years ago I met Michelle Kristensen, who is an expert on food and training, and who charms the whole country on morning TV several times a week. She was my personal trainer for a film role I had to get in shape for and we discovered our mutual hobby – transforming favourite snacks into healthier versions.

Michelle's snack speciality is her healthier version of a Snickers. It is so delicious, and I even prefer this version to a normal store-bought one:

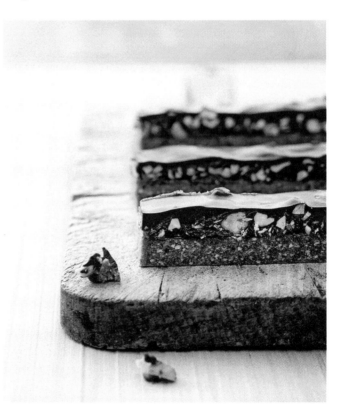

Makes 14

For the base:

250g almonds

150g raisins

4 dates (stones removed)

For the caramel:

16 dates (stones removed)

2 tbsp coconut oil

Pinch of vanilla powder

2 tbsp boiling water

For the topping:

80g salted peanuts, chopped

150g dark chocolate (70 per cent cocoa)

To make the base, process the almonds in a food processor for about 1 minute until they reach a fine texture. Set the almonds aside in a bowl. Process the raisins and dates in a food processor until they form a smooth paste, add the almonds and process the entire mixture. Place the mixture between two pieces of greaseproof paper and, using a rolling pin, roll it out until you have a square that is 1 cm thick.

To make the caramel, blend the dates, coconut oil, vanilla and water in a blender until it becomes a uniform caramel-like mass. It shouldn't be runny, but should hang easily on a spoon. Add a few additional dates or put it in the fridge if it is too runny – just be aware that it solidifies quickly.

Smooth the caramel over the base and sprinkle with chopped peanuts. Melt the chocolate in a bain-marie and pour it over the caramel. Let the chocolate cool, then cut the mixture into 14 pieces and place them in the fridge.

The bars can also be frozen. Yum!

How to Bring *Hygge*
to the Dining Table

- Think like *Lady and the Tramp* – backyard, low-key, simple, good food, a candle, and lots of love and togetherness.
- Invite friends to *hygge* in your home. Cook or bake something simple or make it easy for yourself and let everybody bring something to share.
- Make your own personal book with your signature dishes and the recipes that mean *hygge* to you.

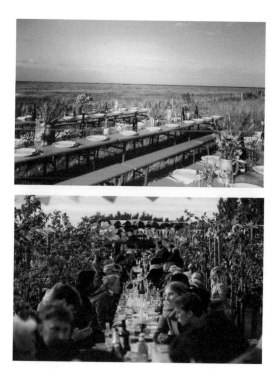

HOW TO BRING *HYGGE* INTO YOUR HOME

– I find hygge inside when nature is raging outside

Twenty-nine-year-old Jakob Nyholm Jessen bought a ramshackle hovel with rats in the attic and mould under the floorboards. But the hovel lay on a scenic site, right next to a forest, a running stream and fields with sheep, so he tore it down and built his own home for his family.

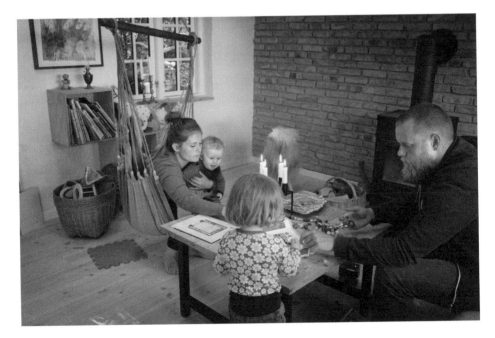

66 Seeking warmth and comfort inside when it's cold and dark outside epitomizes *hygge* for me. I love to be outside, but that's only because I know I can find shelter again when I go inside and shut the door behind me. *Hygge* lies in the contrast, and for me the contrast between outside and inside is greatest when I am close to nature; when darkness is blackest, and there is an absence of street lamps, when the wind is heard sharpest as it shakes the treetops of the forest. The most *hyggelig*, for me, is when I hear the elements raging outside, but I can shut them out and light the fire for heat and light for me and my family.

Therefore, it was a dream come true for me to build my family's home and to build it on a site close to nature. A home where Signe and our children can seek shelter and feel safe and which can be a good backdrop for our lives for many years. Where Niels can learn to crawl, and Agnes read her first words. And where Signe and I can enjoy a glass of red wine in front of the wood-burning stove with our legs up on the sofa.

My thoughts about a home are very much inspired by *The Hobbit*, which was read aloud to me as a child. Their homes were described as secure bases, with soft armchairs, round windows and large storehouses filled with gifts from good friends. Not at all grand.

Signe and I have talked about having a map of the forest up in the living room, so we can draw our favourite forest trails on it. Just like Bilbo did in *The Hobbit*. We also want to mark on the map where we find edible mushrooms in the autumn, so we can remember the good spots for next year. I look forward to the cold winter setting in. Then we put a piece of firewood in the wood-burning stove before we go for a walk in the snowy woods, and when we get home the living room is nice and cosy, and the kids can warm their little hands and noses.**"**

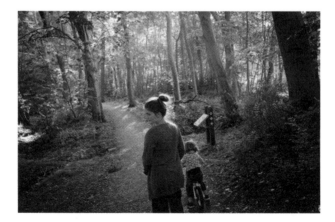

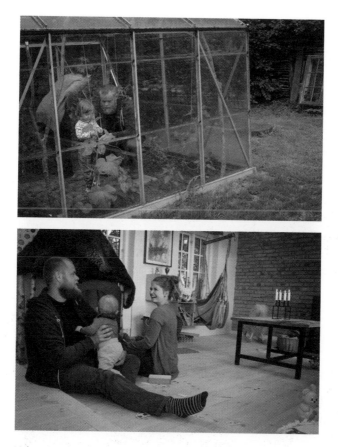

When Signe and I talked about how the rooms in the house were to be distributed, it was important for us to create a kitchen-cum-living-room with the wood-burning stove as the focal point. And it works very well. Signe and I can start the dinner in the kitchen while the kids play on the living-room floor. Although we are all doing our own things, we are still together. Life is lived around the stove.

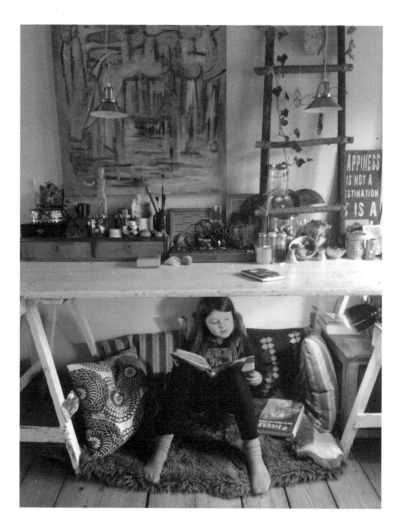

A *hyggelig* home

A *hyggelig* home embraces you and comforts you. It meets you with an uplifting atmosphere and a feeling of belonging. Danes spend quite some time indoors, due to the unpredictable weather, and therefore we put both time and energy into creating a *hyggelig* home.

66 *Hygge* has the wonderful nature of varying from home to home, and often I am surprised how many different places and styles I consider as *hyggelig.*

Hygge is strongly related to feeling safe. The *hygge* comes when you can feel that the person behind the surroundings is completely comfortable with his or her choices, but at the same time isn't afraid of decorating intuitively and trying out new things and ideas.

A home decorated in 'the right way' with things, furniture and aesthetic style chosen exclusively from some kind of formula or specific scheme that is thought to be 'correct', is seldom very *hyggelig.*

In fact, *hygge* grows out of a sincerity in the things you surround yourself with – the settings and framework of your home should reflect the choices you have made regarding your life and your everyday. If you love cooking, guests and food, probably your *hygge* will seep through your kitchen and around the table. In the same way, an art lover's enthusiasm and delight will give the home a different kind of mood and atmosphere according to their chosen aesthetic on display.

The *hygge* of your home will undoubtedly also reflect the time and energy you dedicate to the place. When you put thoughtfulness into how and why you have chosen to surround yourself with particular furniture, objects, art, flowers, knick-knacks, curtains – whatever – then you relax and your guests will see and know you for who you are.99

Christina B. Kjeldsen,
editor and author of several books
on Nordic interior design and lifestyle

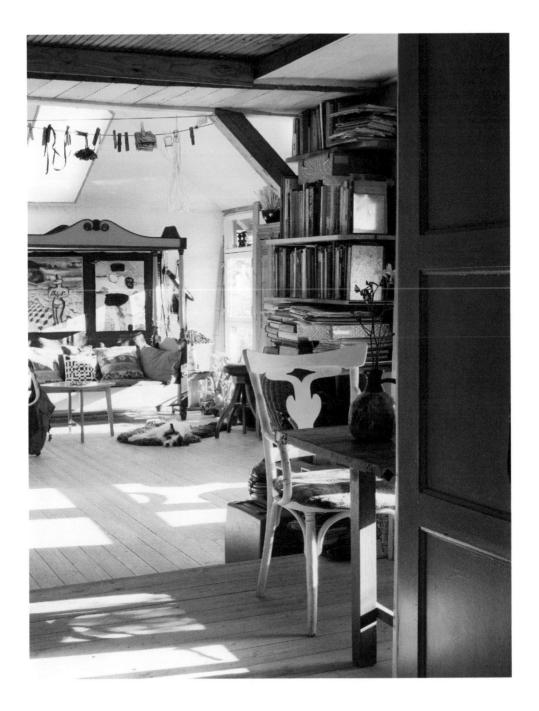

Danish Design

❝ Aesthetics is what tickles the senses and pleases the eye. We thrive in a home we find beautiful, and the aesthetics of it make us take good care of our things. Aesthetics is the pleasure, the sensuality and what makes our surroundings feel special. ❞

Christina B. Kjeldsen

Denmark has a long history of design. With traits of simplicity and functionality, Danish designers such as Arne Jacobsen, Finn Juhl and Poul Henningsen (PH) have made Danish design well-known worldwide. Danish design strives for aesthetics and beauty, but it always has a twist of functionality. The objects are designed to be used, they are not exhibition pieces that no one is allowed to touch. If something is only beautiful, too luxurious and extravagant, it detracts from the relaxed and down-to-earth quality that is a key value in *hygge*.

❝ The PH lamp has an interesting and contemporary cutting-edge design, but as everyone knows, it is built for giving better light. Its appearance is not just superficial design-nonsense to make it unnecessarily beautiful. Oh no, its design directly supports its function: to provide good light. It is an honest lamp; its outer is inseparable from its interior. And when Danish consumers know that, they can live with its beauty. ❞

Jeppe Trolle Linnet, professor of *hygge*

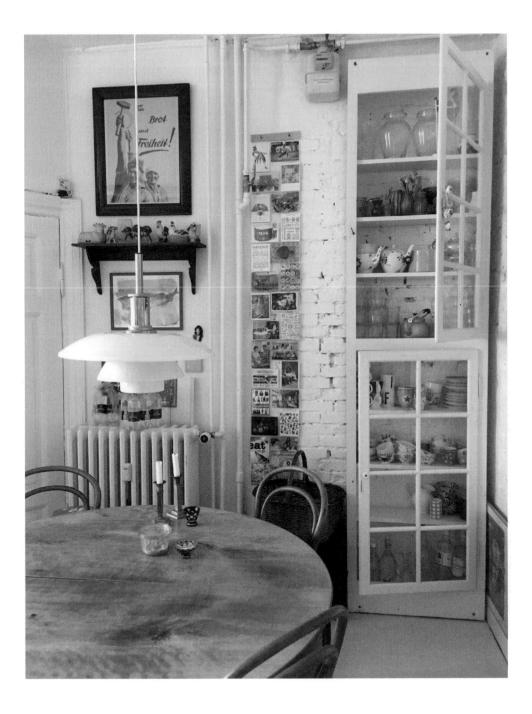

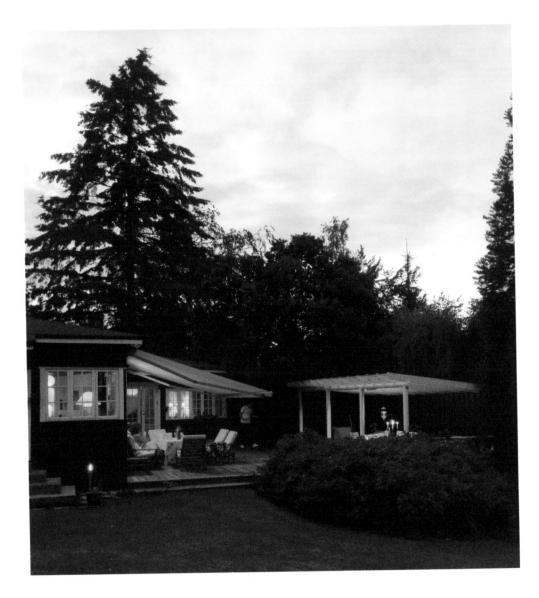

A ROUND TRIP

THROUGH THE

ROOMS OF

THE HOUSE

Hallway

66 The hallway is a room you walk through, a room in between and easy to forget. Nevertheless, it is the very first place that greets you when you come home. Find out what gives you joy to catch sight of when you step inside – a painting from your favourite artist, the colour green or your slippers standing in the hallway, waiting for you to slip into and get comfortable right away. At the same time have an eye on your practical needs. It is neither handy nor *hyggelig* to step directly into a mountain of shoes and coats that blocks your view and restricts your movement. Find functional storage solutions that create space and don't steal too much attention. 99

Christina B. Kjeldsen

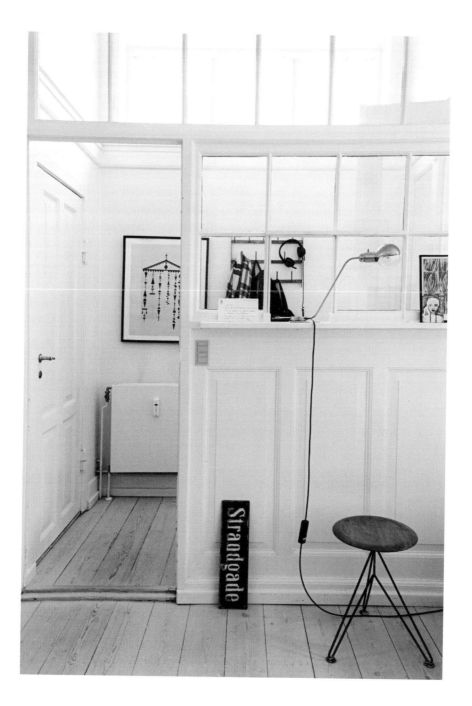

Kitchen

66 From a Scandinavian point of view, *hygge* is also connected to something edible, which naturally sends the kitchen to the top of the *hygge*-barometer.

The kitchen is supposed to be a workshop where you can cook, but if it isn't something you are passionate about, it will probably not be a room you will prioritize. The *hygge* follows the pleasure and interest. Try to transfer what speaks to you especially. If you love baking, then make it easy and inviting for yourself. Have the right tools, baking gear and things that inspire you. If greens, sprouting and plant food make you happy, then make room to immerse yourself in this kind of kitchen life. Have basil, mint and coriander on the windowsill, garlic, chilli and onions in a bowl. Mess is seldom *hyggelig*, unless it is light and pleasant. Clinical surfaces and excessive cleanliness scares you away rather than inviting you in. Kitchens often come as a package deal. Give yours some character and hang up your favourite pots and pans, exhibit tea, tools and decorate the walls with your favourite pictures.

Beware of putting a brand-new kitchen in an old half-timbered house. Respect the architecture and the thoughts behind it, and navigate from there when choosing materials, colours and style. If possible have a small table in the corner with room for people to converse, hang out and keep the chef company. Having a cup of tea or a glass of wine in the off-stage kitchen area can be wonderfully informal and a natural shortcut to a moment of *hygge.* 99

Christina B. Kjeldsen

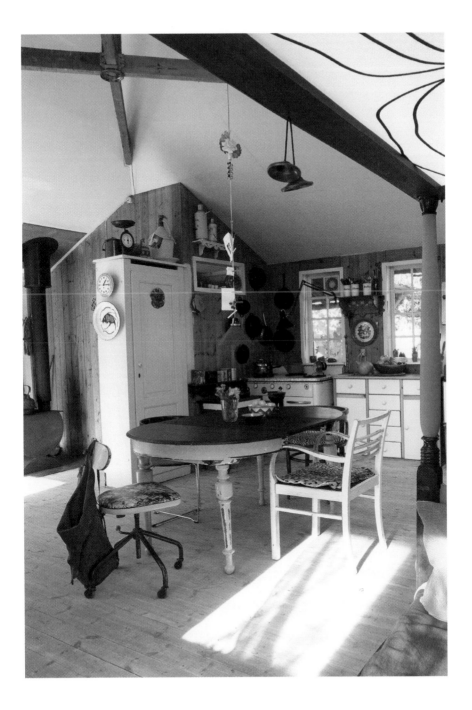

Living Room

66 The living room is often the star turn of the home. From a Scandinavian perspective, materials play a big part when it comes to *hygge*. Wood, folded lampshades of paper, ceramics and stoneware are a part of the Scandinavian style-DNA. We love to surround ourselves with light, Nordic types of wood, just as we have a long tradition of classical furniture design in teak that many of us carry with us as memories from our childhood homes. This brings about the element of recognition that can help define and create the framework for *hygge*. It feels good – it is *hyggelig* – when we recognize pieces of furniture as old friends from the home of our childhood. Many Scandinavians carry this kind of furniture heritage with them due to our history of design, and for a lot of people this helps to create a *hyggelig* and nourishing atmosphere in our homes. If you have a closer look at your own history there will definitely be similar elements you can transfer to your own rooms. What is the unifying point for you – is it the big, big sofa that you grew up with, a special kind of tapestry on the walls or your beloved dresser? 99

Christina B. Kjeldsen

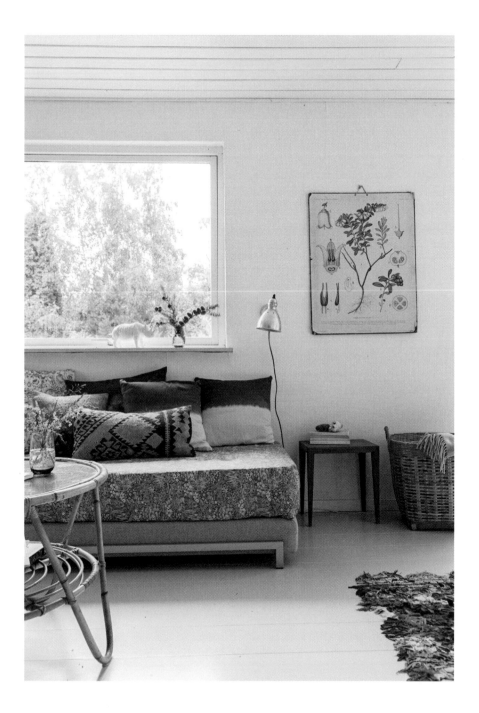

Bathroom

❝ Invite nature into your bathroom with a bathroom table or shelves for storage made of wood, a wicker basket for laundry or a couple of green plants that thrive in the humid climate. And give yourself a little bit of everyday luxury by having an abundance of warm, clean towels in a stack. Make sure the lighting is soft and warm and, yes, a candle is suitable in the bathroom as well as in every other room of the house. Bathrooms allow dwelling. A moment by oneself.❞

Christina B. Kjeldsen

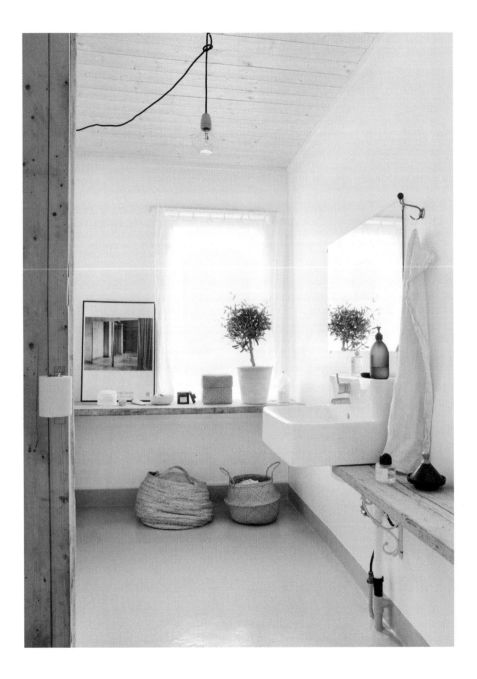

Bedroom

66 This is indeed the most intimate room, the heart of the home. This is where we retreat to, recharge and undress – figuratively and literally speaking. The bedroom should be a room that respects this, so it has to be comforting – really comforting. How you create the atmosphere and the *hygge* here is definitely a question of who you are. If, for example, the colour blue calms you down, then this could be a good colour to dress your bed linen and textiles in. Painting a single wall in the colour you like can also give your bedroom character and depth. Do you have special pieces of art, photos or prints that send you towards sweet dreams? These are what suit your walls. Remember to make space for your special routines – a place for your book, your glass of water, your jewellery, a mirror. If you prefer having things in order, a good organized storage might play a central part for your wellbeing, while a beautiful chair to throw your clothes on would be the optimal solution for others. *Hygge* comes with authenticity, when you decorate your home following your heart – especially in this room, where you are your innermost self. 99

Christina B. Kjeldsen

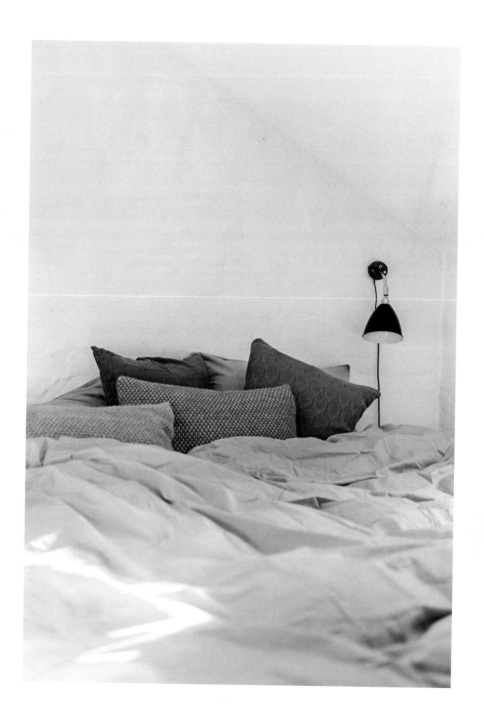

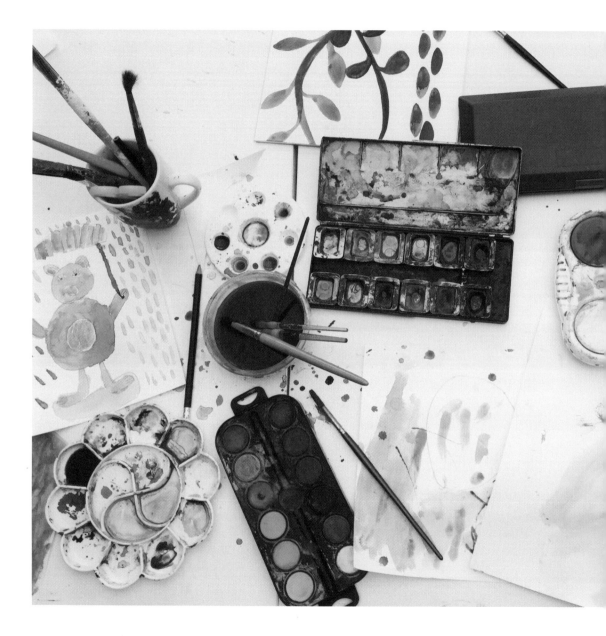

10

TIPS FOR
INSPIRATION

Plants

66 More is more and less is less. This is a good way of thinking when it comes to plants. Many plants together work better than a house plant here and a house plant there. Dedicate one area to being green; perhaps a special table to put your plants on and next to, and to hang more from the ceiling above. In this way you create a vigorous, green area in your home, where plants rule.99

Christina B. Kjeldsen

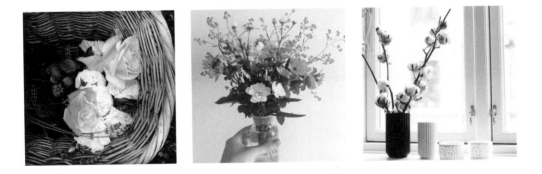

A beautiful bouquet picked in a field or flowery branches from the apple tree in your garden can make a corner bloom. Or why not go with a cotton branch with soft buds that can last for years.

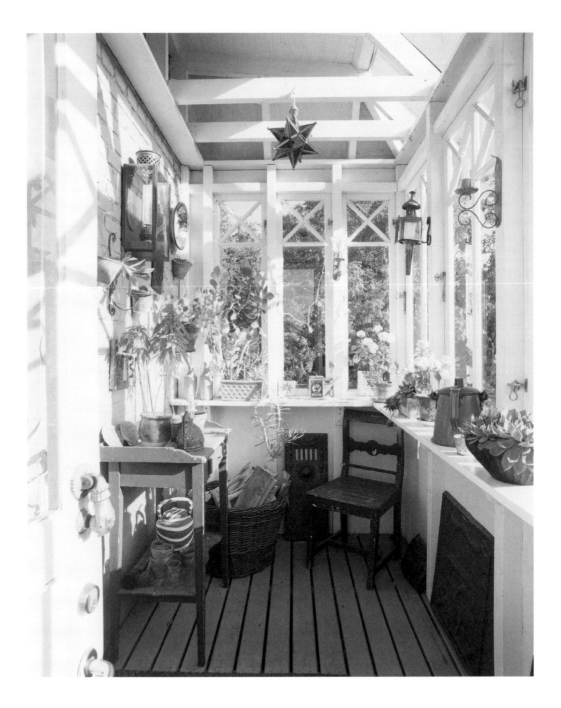

Corners

When you decorate your home, make room for charging stations – not only for your phone or computer, but for yourself and your family. Corners give us a feeling of being safe and can be a great place to recharge. Place an armchair in a corner with a couple of soft cushions and a blanket. Have a lamp and a small table next to you, so you can lose yourself in a good book with a cup of tea and a snack on the side.

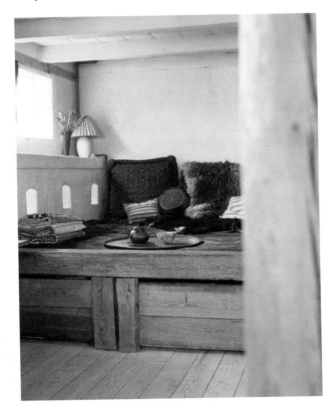

Presents and heirlooms

Sometimes we hardly take notice of the things we surround ourselves with, but when we take a closer look some of them tell stories about us and contain memories from special times spent with dear ones. Being aware of these stories adds meaning and *hygge* to our surroundings.

Treasuring our presents and heirlooms is valuing their story.

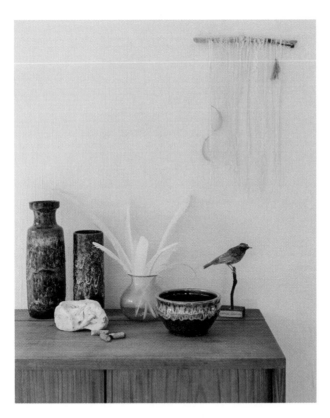

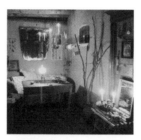

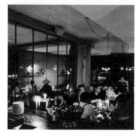

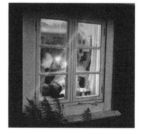

Lighting

In the northern hemisphere we try to get as much daylight into our homes as possible, but due to the climate, we depend on artificial light during the daytime for six to eight months of the year. Therefore, what light and lamps we surround ourselves with at home and at work is no trivial matter. Light is vital for our well-being, says the Danish light architect Asger Bay Christensen, who shares his best tricks for creating *hygge*-light.

" **Choose an incandescent bulb or a warm LED diode for your light source.** For those of us who live in a cold country, *hygge* light is warm light. The colour temperature of light is measured in degrees Kelvin, and a Kelvin degree of 2,700 gives off a yellow/orange tinge, what I call a warm light, and that is *hygge* for me and, I believe, for most Danes.

Make small pools of light: have a minimum of two lamps in each room – even in small rooms. Turn off the overhead light and create small light pools instead. Have a well-shielded hanging lamp over your table so that the light does not shine directly into your eyes, but is focused down on the table, thereby lighting only the table. Do the same over the coffee table and above your books on the shelf. Having a dimmer switch is also a way to adjust the light according to your needs and mood. "

Candles

❝ I am certain of one thing: If there is something Danes don't want to run short of, it is toilet paper and candles. Luckily you can get both in even the smallest shop.❞

Roger Beale, Brit living in Denmark, in Politiken

Within the EU, Denmark uses the most kilograms of stearin per capita – 5.79 kilos of candles are used by each Dane, every year.

❝ I light a candle as the first thing I do when I come home after a day's work. It sends me the message that it is time to dwell and relax. I also always bring candles with me when I travel; then I am always sure that I can make myself a *hyggelig* time, no matter where I go or what hotel I stay in.❞

Tilde Vengsgaard, Randers

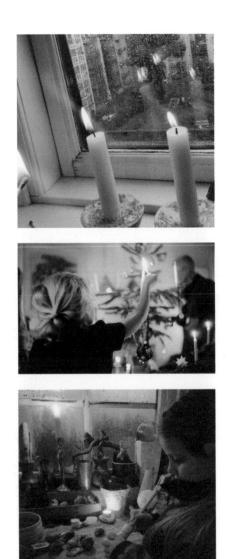

Books

These naturally contain stories and sometimes their cover, material, where they came from and the places they have been also tell a story of their own. The books we have tell a story of who we are. Old books from your parents or grandparents, books found on vacation, favourite books, books from your childhood bedtime stories or the one you read the first time you were madly in love.

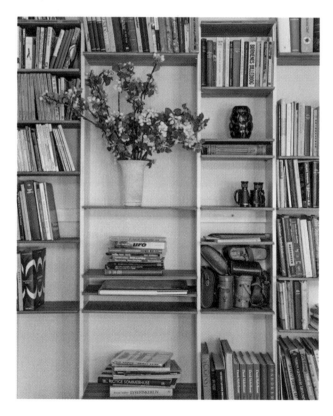

Recycle

Re-using pallets, jars, boxes and pipes adds patina to our surroundings. Clean a used jar and turn it into a drinking glass or a vase for flowers you picked from the hedgerow on your way home. Use apple boxes for storing books or as a table and old pipes as a clothes rack.

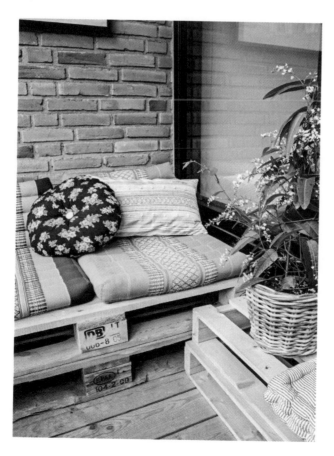

Music

66 The musical take on hygge is often misunderstood as people believe that you have to go back to a brown, kitschy 70's kind of sound and avoid too much musical content. That is not how it is.

Hygge is the soft, warm feeling of peace of mind. A nest of togetherness and undisturbed presence. Something very fine that can be served in a thousand different ways, but always has togetherness and presence at its core.

Here are ten tracks that all contain warm togetherness, content and something essential. Ten tracks that automatically and in a subtle way put you in a hyggelig mood, where you want to spend time with other people; sit close, right now and for a long while.99

- Morten Lindberg, a.k.a. Master Fatman,
Danish DJ and legendary radio host

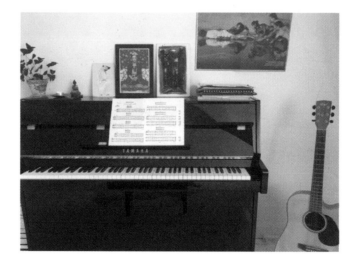

138

The *Hygge* Playlist –
by Master Fatman

1.
I'm Still in Love With You / Marcia Aitken

2.
As She Walked Away / Brother Jack McDuff

3.
Lua, Lua, Lua, Lua / Gal Costa

4.
What Are You Doing the Rest of Your Life? / Bill Evans

5.
Besoka On Salsa / Manu Dibango

6.
Samba Saravah / Pierre Barouh

7.
The Sewing Machine / The Sea and Cake

8.
O Rio Para Trás / Celso Fonseca

9.
I Wish You Love / Blossom Dearie

10.
Ain't No Sunshine / Sivuca

Souvenirs

Bringing souvenirs home with us from travels leaves traces of where we have been. You can go for more functional souvenirs – a pasta machine from your trip to Sicily, wooden kitchen utensils from an ironmonger in southern France or a soap dispenser made of Icelandic volcanic stone. Don't be afraid of the cliché of souvenirs; if a mini version of the Eiffel Tower reminds you of an unforgettable trip to Paris, bring it back with you and enjoy how the memories follow suit.

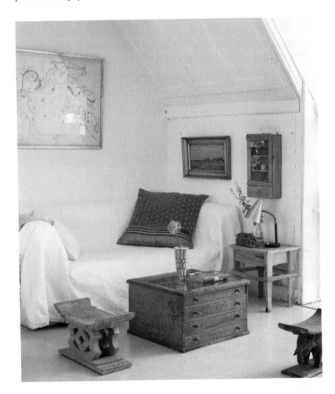

Mix and Match

Mixing old and new is a way of balancing a home. Mix the old antique dresser you inherited with a brand-new lamp you find beautiful, a chair from the flea market and a picture your friend painted for you.

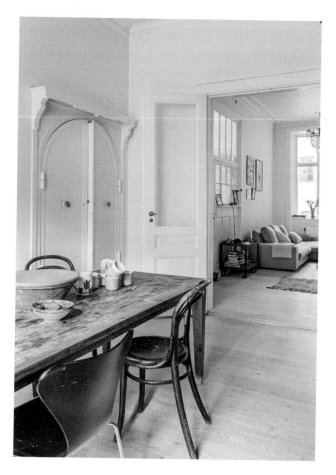

Working Space

We spend a lot of time at work, so why not make it a bit *hyggelig*? Having a *hyggelig* atmosphere is not only restricted to your home area – you can easily bring the ideas mentioned in this chapter with you to work. Design a workplace that allows you to do your best in the most enjoyable way.

Personality – *Set up a mood board as inspiration with photos from wonderful holidays, a beautiful picture from Hammershøi or Monet, a drawing from your niece or a newspaper cartoon that makes you giggle.*

Tidy – *Get some elbow room by getting rid of papers that you don't need any more and find good storage solutions for the rest. Have boxes in bright colours and patterns and recycle an old porcelain vase for your pens and pencils.*

Flow – *Having good lighting and life on our desk is inspiring to our work flow. Make sure you have proper lighting that hits the desk and your papers directly, without spreading out. Have candles and fresh flowers or plants around you. And don't forget to have your favourite mug by your side, reminding you to take an enjoyable break with your colleagues.*

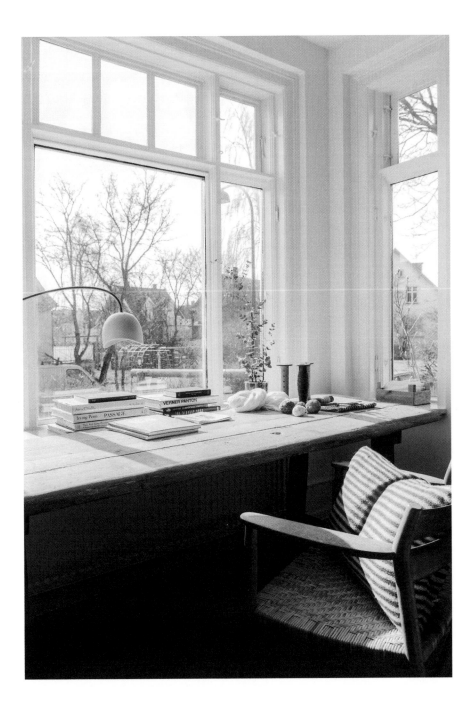

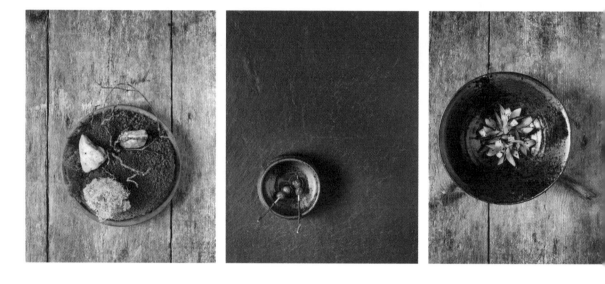

Hygge and Honesty in the Michelin League

With tools such as light, materials and colours, the Danish interior architects Signe Bindslev Hansen and Peter Bundgaard Rützou create atmospheres of *hygge* in some of Denmark's most acclaimed restaurants. On the basis of their work in world-famous Nordic food restaurant Noma, they give an insight into how they help *hygge* evolve:

> ❝ *Hygge* has a complex nature and succeeding in creating a '*hyggelig* atmosphere' is about succeeding in passing on a feeling of belonging, feeling embraced and to some extent recognized.
>
> When we started the project with Noma, the chef of the restaurant, René Redzepi, gave us only one brief. He wanted no artificial, conceptual filter between the guest and the actual food experience. He wanted honest, one-to-one – no gimmicks, no pop. And it became our aim to try to get as seamless an integration between aesthetics and function as possible. ❞

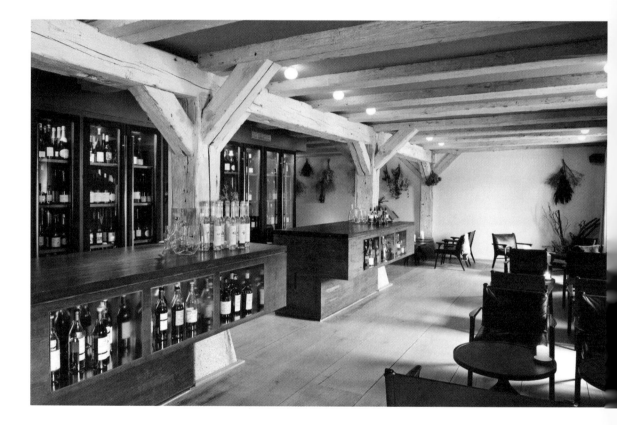

Materials

66 All our projects start from the definition of the material palette and we have always had a deep passion for organic materials, such as variations of woods, stones, wools, linens, leathers and metals. This was our initial approach to the Noma project too, which felt perfectly in line with the organic and philosophical approach of René Redzepi and the Noma Kitchen. The great thing about organic materials is that, if you treat them right, they have the ability to age well. How they carry the story of being used over time is the best example of bringing soul, authenticity, attachment and a sense of belonging – qualities like these are closely attached to the phenomenon of *hygge*, we believe.99

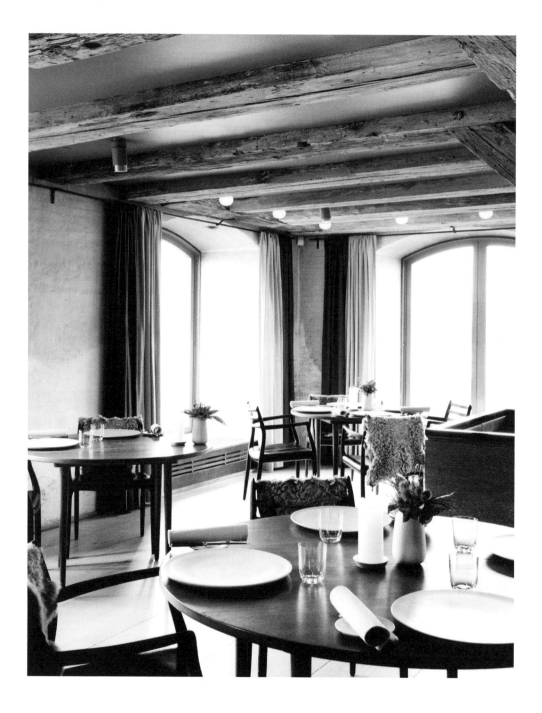

Lighting

66 First of all, we wanted to allow the outside light to blend into the space – when useful. Therefore, we put in both sheers and more solid curtains to give the staff the scope to adjust them. We generally wished for an intense, soft, low-lit lighting and atmosphere and we chose a soft overall simple ceiling light fixture with the option to dim to almost nothing. That secured us a great homely feel – the feeling of not being exposed.

Lastly, we love the element of candles and oil lamps, which we have also used in Noma in various ways. 99

Colours

66 The colours originate more or less from the colours of the materials. We like that the colour of an organic material most often originates from its history – it tells you about the process it has been through, about the way it has been treated and where it comes from. At the same time the colour of a natural material is strengthened by its basic characteristics of texture, pattern and depth. We also think it is important to remember that when we have finished our part of the job, the space still needs to be able to welcome a lot of other elements before it's fully completed – the beauty of all the colourful food, which should be central to the experience, and all the people inhabiting the room – therefore we generally like to keep the colours in soft, chalky and dusted nuances. 99

Open kitchen

66 The open kitchen brings everybody closer, creating intimacy and a sense of home. And not only can the guest see the chefs and the beautiful scenery of the food and kitchen, it is just as important to allow the chefs to feel fuelled by the energy in the restaurant and the guests' reactions to the food. 99

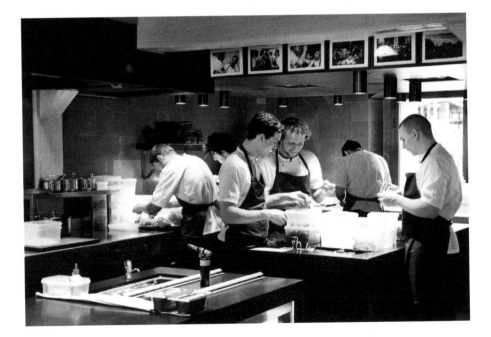

She Creates Atmospheres for a Living

As a set designer, Mia Stensgaard creates spaces for specific atmospheres: atmospheres of coldness, of reconciliation and of pure *hygge*. She is behind the production design for the Danish award-winning television series *Arvingerne* (*The Legacy*) and the absurd film comedy *Mænd og Høns* (*Men and Chicken*). Based on photos from these two productions, Mia Stensgaard shares with us how she evokes an atmosphere of *hygge*.

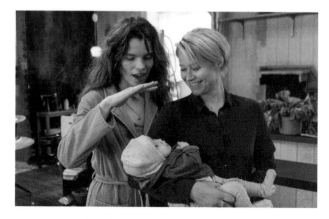

Photo from *The Legacy* by Per Arnesen

Mia Stensgaard:

❝ A dressing gown is an intimate garment often worn only in domestic situations and in situations where you feel safe. In a dressing gown you are vulnerable and not prepared to face the outside world yet. Only those people to whom you are closest see you in your dressing gown.

The pink dressing gown here recurs in most seasons of *The Legacy*. It belonged to the main characters' mother, and the adult children take turns to wear it during the first and second seasons. This signifies that despite intrigue, cruelty and hostility, they are connected.

The family's youngest daughter, Signe, has not been a part of the family for many years, as she was given up for adoption when she was little. In this photo, from a scene in the second season, she is wearing the dressing gown, and for me it's the most *hyggelig* way to show that she has been initiated as a full member of the family.❞

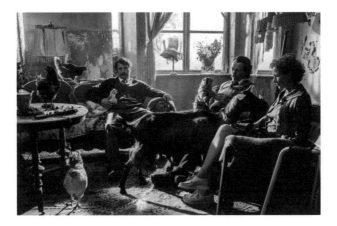

Photo from *Men and Chicken* by Rolf Konow

❝ I work on the assumption that *hygge* thrives best in spaces that invite you in without making you feel that you need to behave in a certain way when there. When you enter a room where you are immediately nervous about leaving fingerprints on a newly polished glass table, *hygge* is restricted.

But if there's a red wine stain on the wall or cracks in the floors, it signals that here life is lived with all the little accidents it can bring. Here you can just be, relax, *hygge* yourself – and if you break something, then we can just fix it again.

I worked to create such spaces for the comedy *Men and Chicken*.❞

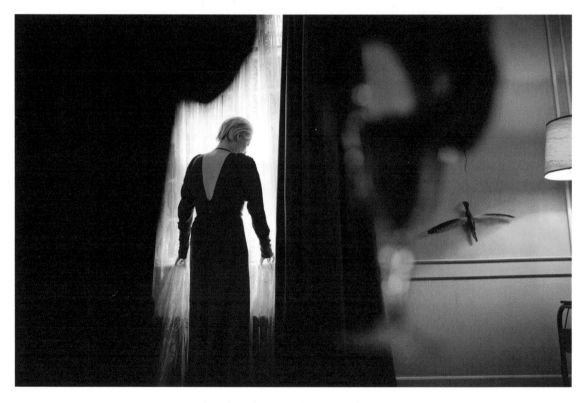

Photo from *The Legacy* by Martin Lehmann

❝❝ For me *hygge* equals community. When I create a space where *hygge* can occur, I often include visible reminders of a community in the room.

The driftwood with wings on the wall is supposed to be a gift that the TV show's main characters made as children for their mother. Gifts like this are found throughout the entire house and tell us that the house was once the setting for a family with room for both children and art.

In fact the driftwood has its own little personal history. It is actually my own father and son who are behind this creation.

I was raised by a pair of art teacher parents in the 1970s – and the concept of ' finding forms' was a large part of their teaching. The driftwood with wings is a good example of this concept: when you are finding forms, you can find various components in nature, for example, which are each their own thing, but which, when they are put together, become something new.❞❞

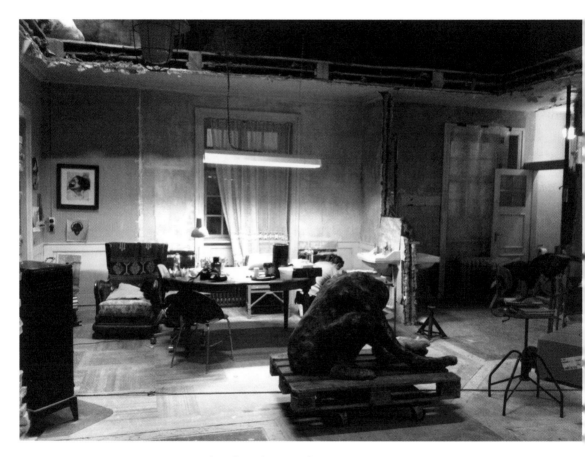

Photo from *The Legacy* by Mia Stensgaard

❝ The mother's house is an artist's house, and I wanted the scenes at home to ooze a feeling of Santa's workshop. Here, the design of a piece of art has taken place right in the middle of the living room, surrounded by everyday pursuits. It tells a story that this is a home where desire, ideas, chores and activities merge.

The right atmosphere and the community are prioritized over aesthetics, order and standards.

In my own life I also find that when I dare to relinquish control and relax standards and order, I find the most *hygge*.

In Denmark, we have a culture of inviting people home, and when I invite good friends to a party at home, it is pure *hygge*, for me, when I am able to relinquish control and let the guests come before the actual event to help with the preparations; in the same way, I often find that the after-party ends up being more *hyggelig* than the planned party itself. During the event both guests and hosts have a habit of keeping to standards and adhering to unspoken expectations. But gold is found at the edges. It is at the pre-party that we sit together round the kitchen table, twenty people, where there is effectively only seating for eight. And, likewise, it is at the after-party that we laugh because one person has ended up with a black eye, while another has fallen head-over-heels in love, and none of it was planned, but it happened, and now here we are. ❞

HYGGE

THROUGHOUT

THE YEAR

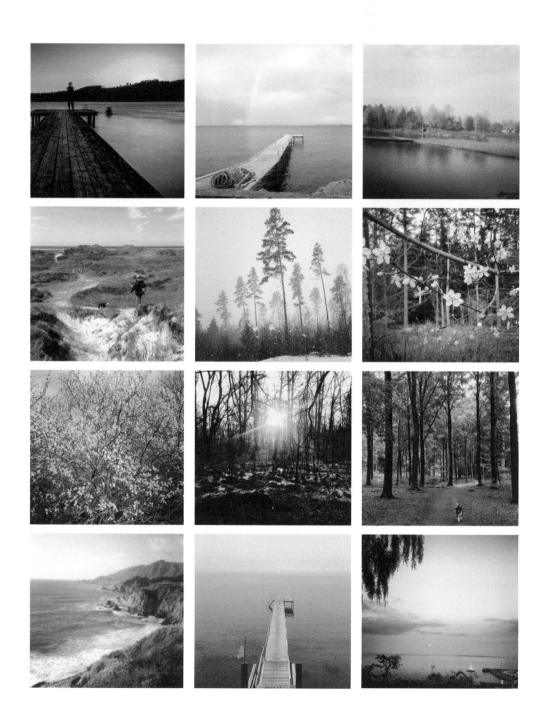

❝ I associate *hygge* with both light and dark. In winter, in the pitch-black months, everything has to be done indoors, and you have to make it *hyggelig* to keep going. So you gather in front of the hearth, packed in blankets and surrounded by candles, and move closer together and draw the curtains as protection against the night outside. And when the light slowly returns in February, March and April, you climb out of your cave more and more; sitting stubbornly, half frozen, on a pavement café one early evening in spring, drinking beer, huddled against the wind, but you continue, and the evenings are wonderfully *hyggelig*, in a weird way, full of unity against the cold and a feeling of victory; we did it again.

When the summer really comes, when the light in June and July never really disappears, *hygge* moves out to the coasts. Families take to the countryside, camping behind inverted boats on the beach, you meet people you have not seen all winter and gossip about what has happened since last year. You spend your days reading books and walking lazily around until it starts to rain. Then you retreat indoors, bake fruit cakes and read Donald Duck comics, but as soon as the sun peeks out again, you move out on to the terrace for a good lunch with rye bread and beer, go on fishing trips, bathe and live life on the beach during those few days of the year that it is possible. The life that takes place there is the *hyggeligste* and happiest that I know of, and I take that sense of community that arises out of that pure summer euphoria with me under the blankets throughout the winter. ❞

Amalie Laulund Trudsø

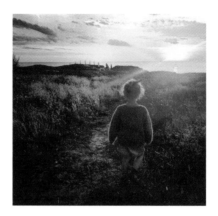

ACTIVITIES

ALL YEAR ROUND

Due to the big changes in seasons, the *hygge* changes character
depending on what time of year it is:

Springtime

When winter has held me tight for more than the estimated three months, and I have bravely lit candles and kept up the good spirit indoors, and I look down on the ground and see the first snowdrop, I realize how much I have waited for this moment. The first sign that spring and light are on their way.

It is a beautiful season that coaxes you outdoors again after months spent *hygge*-caving. It lures you out with flowers and green buds on the trees and the promise of a new beginning. Nature is blooming and so is the mood of most of the population.

To me this time of seasonal *hygge* involves moving outside again: enjoying a cup of coffee in a streak of sunlight, picking snowdrops and anemones and putting them in a vase, and enjoying the two weeks of immensely beautiful cherry blossom in April.

This season also has many traditions and minor holidays that are worth celebrating.

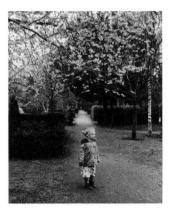

Secret snowdrop letters (gækkebrev)

A month before Easter, friends and family send out small letters to each other signed with just a little dot for each letter in the sender's name. If the receiver can't guess who it is from, he owes the sender a chocolate egg. This tradition is an old Danish custom that dates all the way back to the eighteenth century when young lovers would send paper cuttings to one another.

How to make a snowdrop letter

Take a piece of writing paper. Fold the top right corner down, to form a square. Cut the excess bottom part off so you now have a triangle. Fold the triangle twice more into a smaller triangle. Cut off the top (the part where the ends meet) to make the letter round. Now it is time to be creative – make cuts on either side of the triangle. Unfold it, and write your verse; don't forget to write your name in dots. Put it in an envelope together with a dried snowdrop flower and send it off.

Verse for a snowdrop letter:

Snowdrop, snowdrop, snowdrop fine
Omen true and hope divine
From the heart of winter brings
A delightful glimpse of spring.
Guess my name I humbly beg
Your reward – an Easter egg.
Let these puzzling dots proclaim
Every letter of my name . . . . .

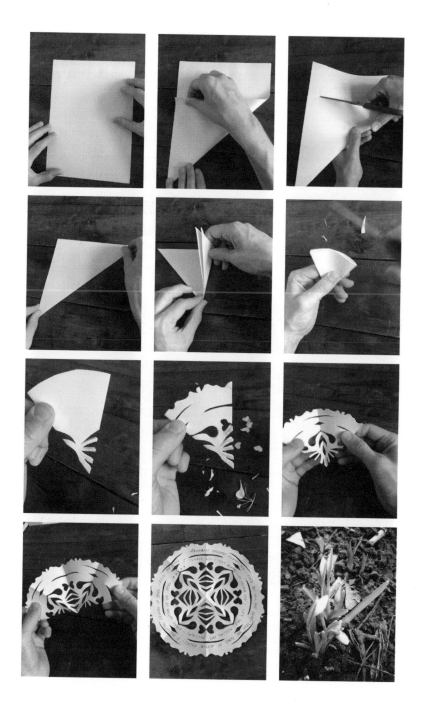

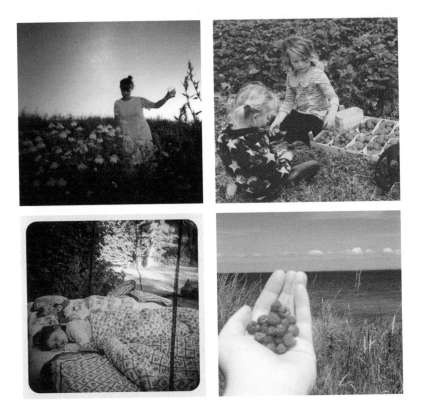

Summertime

Summertime is holiday time, potter about in slippers time, togetherness time. Time for having long breakfasts on the terrace in the mornings, and having a barbecue or lighting a bonfire in the long and light summer evenings.

Summer-*hygge* also involves canning and preserving all the great tastes of the season, so you can still have the taste of summer even in the depths of winter. I make pickled tomatoes or onions, jam from fruits and berries – or this great elderflower cordial:

SUMMER IN A GLASS — ELDERFLOWER CORDIAL

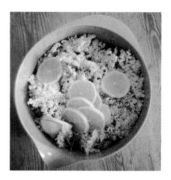

Whenever you have guests over, expected or unexpected, a glass of elderflower lemonade is always a treat. It is homemade and refreshing. Mix the cordial with sparkling or still water, or perhaps add it to some sparkling wine.

Keep it in the fridge or give the bottles as a gift.

The wonderful thing about elderflower is that it grows in the wild, and you have to go on a little expedition to find it.

Cut the elderflowers off with a pair of scissors. Choose the fresh ones that are not brown yet, as this will affect the quality of the cordial.

**Makes approx.
1.5 litres**

20–30 elderflower blossoms

2 organic lemons

2 tbsp citric acid (If you don't have
this, don't worry. It acts as a
preservative that conserves the
cordial. If you don't add it, you
– unfortunately – have to drink it all
within a week . . .)

650g sugar (perhaps cane sugar)

1.2 litres boiling water

Rinse and clean the blossoms and put them in a big pot or bowl
with a lid. Rinse the lemons and slice them. Add them to the pot.
Mix the citric acid with the sugar and dissolve it in the boiling
water. Pour the resulting cordial over the flowers and lemons,
then put the lid on and put it in the fridge for four days.

Pour the elderflower cordial through a sieve then pour it into
clean, sterilized bottles. Mix with water or wine and enjoy.

Tip:

Put the cordial into ice-cube bags and put them in the freezer.
Add one or two to still or sparkling water. This is a great way to
make a glass of ice-cold elderflower lemonade on hot summer
days – or on any day when you long for a taste of summer.

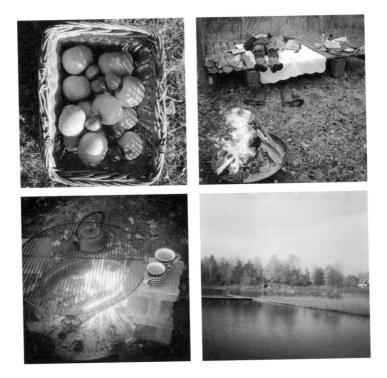

Autumn

From the end of September, I start to prepare myself for hibernation time again. I make sure that my home is well-stocked with candles and take my knitted sweaters down from the top shelf. Autumn is my favourite time of year. Going for a walk in the forest on a blue and bright October day, looking at the beautiful red-brown-orange shades of the trees and kicking the crisp leaves is one of the things I love the most in autumn. When evening starts to fall and the darkness is creeping in, I head back to my home, longing for warmth. Autumn is time to be indoors, to indulge and immerse myself in small projects, books and cooking food for hours on the stove.

'Room for guests', 'soft lighting' and 'a little accompanying snack' are my keywords when I wish to create a *hyggelig* time indoors. The following projects will help you invite the Autumn *hygge* into your home. They are kindly shared with us by the three girls behind the Danish do-it-yourself book *Homesick DIY*.

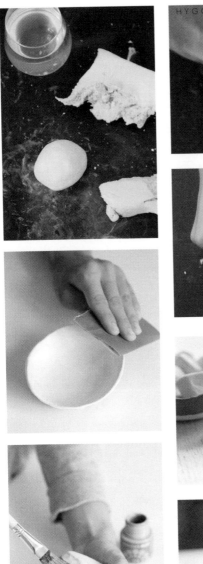
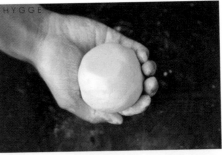
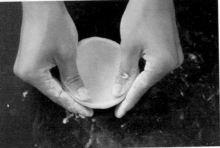
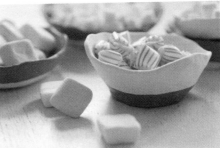
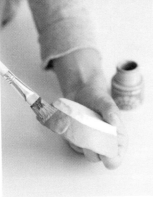
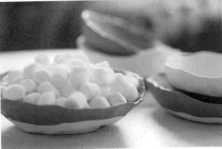

A UNIQUE HOBBY-CLAY BOWL

Hobby clay is a cheap and easy material to work with and it has a nice ceramic look once it has air-dried. Here we've used it to make a bowl and its 'handmade-ness' just adds to its beauty. The irregular form of each bowl is all part of its charm. You can use your unique bowl for decoration, for your jewellery or for your keys. Or, if you give it a coat of environmentally friendly varnish, you can also use it to serve yummy pink marshmallows and other nibbles.

What you need:

Hobby clay

Water

Paintbrush

Fine sandpaper

Hobby varnish

Knead a lump of clay and form it into a ball. It is good to use white hobby clay as it has a nice, natural colour. Smooth out the clay and form it from the middle, pulling out with your thumb, until you reach your desired bowl shape. Be as light as possible with your fingertips if you'd like the bowl to have a thinner edge. Wet your fingertips with water and apply it to the bowl to achieve a smoother finish, to round off edges and to remove as many fingerprints as possible after shaping the bowl.

Let the bowl air dry. This takes about one to two days, depending on the clay and the thickness of the bowl. Always read the instructions on the packet.

You can leave the bowl as it is or you can polish the edges with fine sandpaper to soften them. Only the limits of your imagination restrict the colours and patterns you can use to decorate your bowl. If you want to use the bowl for foodstuffs, remember to coat it in an environmentally friendly hobby varnish afterwards.

Fill the bowl with your favourite sweets and enjoy a *hyggelig* evening curled up on the sofa.

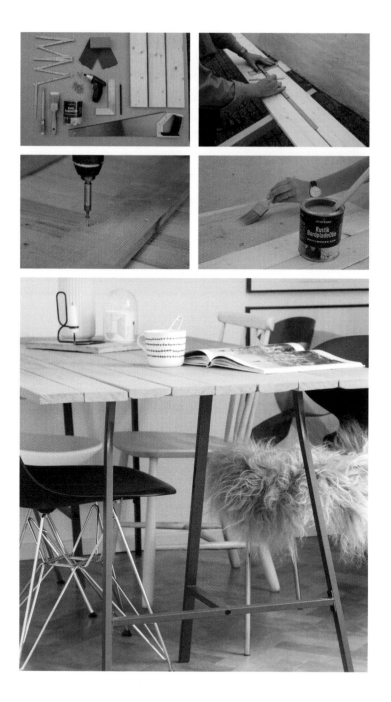

DIY TABLE

To build your own rustic plank table is not at all difficult – and it's budget-friendly. This plank table measures 90cm x 165cm and is suitable for four people, but you can easily make a table to suit your needs.

What you need:

8 planks for the tabletop

1 extra plank, cut in two, to lie across the 8 planks above and hold them together

Saw

Carpenter's measure

Carpenter's square

Pencil

32 flat-head wood screws

Sandpaper, fine and coarse (or an electric sander)

Paintbrush

Wood stain

2 table trestles

Measure the length of the 8 planks and saw them so they are all the same length. Saw the extra plank into two pieces of wood, so they are a little shorter than the width of the table, but are still long enough to lie across all the planks. Sand the planks with the coarse sandpaper and then with the fine one, or with a sander. Sand all surfaces, especially along the edges, where people will sit.

Line the planks up with each other, and lie them with the tabletop side face down. Now place the two shorter pieces of wood across the planks at each end and screw them into place, using screws long enough to pass through both the wood and the planks – but not so long that they break through the tabletop surface. Try to press the planks together as tightly as possible to avoid gaps between the planks in the finished tabletop. Vacuum clean the tabletop for sawdust and wipe it with a damp cloth. Now the tabletop is ready to be stained. We used a grey stain to achieve a rustic look. Always read the instructions and follow the recommended drying time.

When the tabletop is completely dry, you can place it on table trestles, such as those available from IKEA. The tabletop can just rest on the trestles, though we screwed ours on securely.

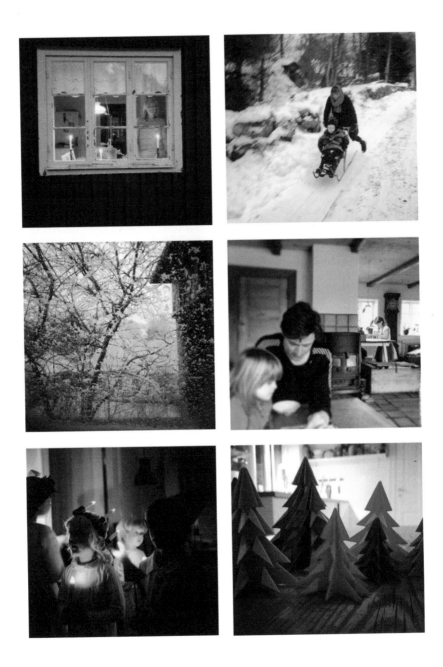

Wintertime

It's time to feel utterly good about gathering on the sofa with family and friends, watching a TV show, playing games, reading, talking, eating simmer food and lighting candles.

This also is the season for making homemade Christmas decorations, baking, meeting each other around mulled wine and pancake puffs, and celebrating St Lucy's Day on 13 December, when choirs parade with candles and sing the Lucia song. Having a string of lights ensures a good atmosphere even when Christmas is over:

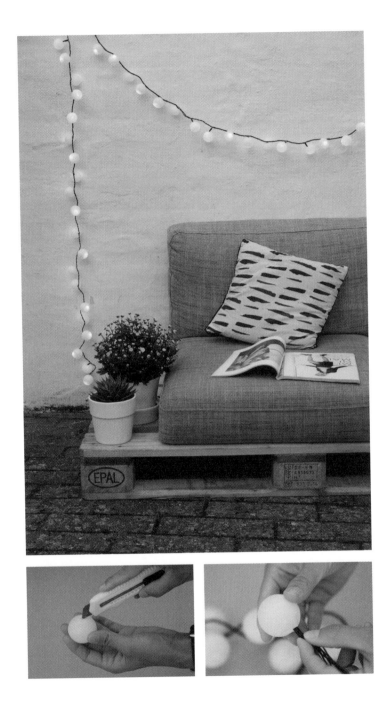

HYGGE
LIGHTS

A string of lights creates the finest glow and a *hyggelig* atmosphere. For this project, we spiced up the classic, boring string of lights with something as ordinary as table-tennis balls to achieve a softer light. It creates *hygge* and a nice atmosphere when darkness falls, wherever you place it – outside or inside, in your favourite corner or wound round the handrail of your terrace.

Make an incision in each table-tennis ball. Try not to cut the joins of the table-tennis balls, as they could break.

Push each of the bulbs from the string of lights firmly through the incisions in the balls. Try to fix any dents or bulges that occur as you press into the balls.

What you need:

A string of lights (LED, so the bulbs do not overheat)

Table-tennis balls (as many as there are bulbs on the string)

A craft knife

Traditions

Whether it is inviting the same group of friends for New Year's Eve every year or celebrating your birthday in the garden, year after year, traditions bring back memories and bind people together.

I have a friend who gathers all her friends for the nowadays little-known Danish tradition Kyndelmisse, in February. It is an old Christian holiday, Candle Mass, celebrating that half the winter is over. We meet late afternoon and bake pancakes together. When the pancakes are all round and ready, we enjoy them at the table set with lighted candles. Naturally.

Why not have a look in your own calendar; go on a search for forgotten holidays or old traditions worthy of a little renaissance.

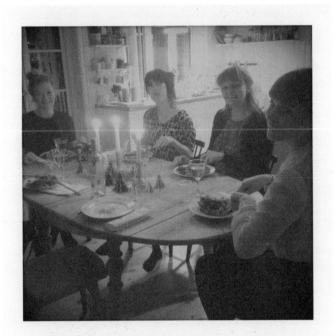

Kyndelmisse, February 2nd, 2014.

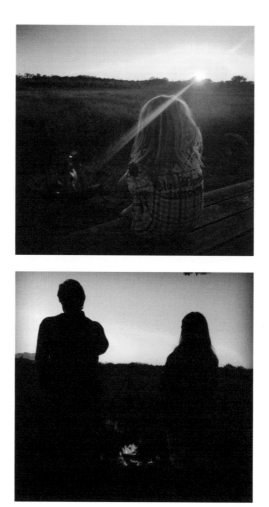

Margrethe lives in the northern part of Jutland with her husband and two children, and since she was a child her family have celebrated an evening called Walpurgis, another occasion that very few Danes celebrate:

❝ On Saturday we celebrated Walpurgis evening (the last evening in April). Some years we have had a garden full of children and adults. But, this year, it was just the four of us. We had an easy morning, sitting at the breakfast table, *hygg*-ing ourselves and talking about why we celebrate Walpurgis, and how I had celebrated it with my parents when I was a child. It brought back wonderful memories of spring evenings with bonfires, games and warm pancakes. The children love to hear those stories. We spent the evening, as per tradition, by the fire. I sat there immersing myself in conversation with my husband, Morten, about everything that we dream of and work towards realizing for us as a family, while the children played nearby. We stayed there by the fire until it got dark – until we all ended up under the same blanket as the fire burnt out – another *hyggelig* night to remember. And I thought how privileged I was to be able to sit there with my family. That I have the opportunity to do so makes me humble. ❞

Margrethe Sønderlund Andersen,
Northern Jutland

Hygge and Time Off

Holiday time is winding down. But you don't necessarily have to travel to the end of the world to experience quality time and *hygge*. Often it is right in front of our noses, or only a short jaunt away. Retreating to an allotment house, a summer house, a ramshackle old farm in Sweden are all *hyggelig* ways in which Danes unwind and relax from everyday life.

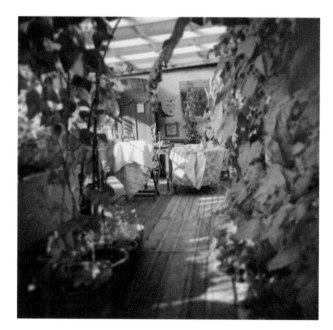

Summer House

The sun is low in the sky now and has coloured every-thing a warm orange, the smallest ridges in the sand casting long shadows behind them. We're allowed to bathe in the evening. For once no one says anything about wet hair and colds, and we just throw off our clothes and run out into the glistening water. When we come back again, our teeth are rattling, we can hardly pull our warm jumpers over our heads because of shaking hands. My plait is dripping wet and leaves a wet trail like a river down my back. The fire has been burning for a while now, the embers have grown and have become flames in twilight's beginning. I sit with my mother, who barely has time to remove the French café glass of red wine before I knock it over the blankets; she puts her arms round me and shakes her head at the wet hair. The heat from the fire lights up our faces, making all their features clearly visible. When a moment is calm, when a single minute or two is quiet from all the adults' talk about the old days, a kind of New Year glides in and settles imperceptibly around us. The lighthouse on Nekselø flashes rhyth-mically, the headland out there only a silhouette against the still-bright sky. When, much later, we walk home along the dark beach path, afraid of stepping on slugs with bare feet, I am certain: winter can come, we will survive.

From *Sommerhus* by Amalie Laulund Trudsø

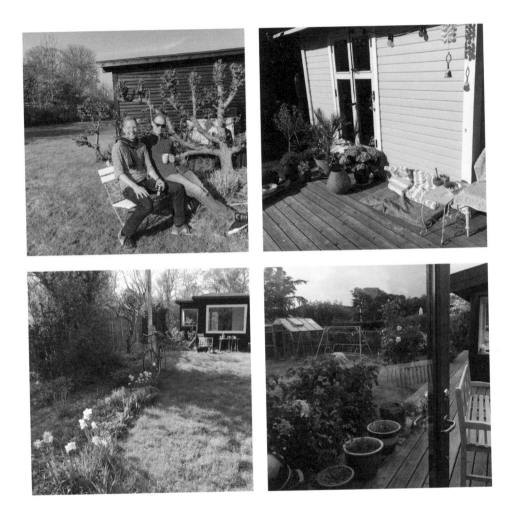

The Allotment House and Garden

66 My family has an allotment fifteen minutes from Copenhagen. It is a simple house, small kitchen, small living room and small bed. Actually everything is small – except for the garden where we have grown flowers, rows of herbs and some vegetables in raised beds. I come out here when I need to focus without distractions, or when I just need to unwind. I mow the lawn, enjoy a beer on the veranda, read a book or prepare apple seedlings. I love to cook and being able to grow my own herbs and vegetables makes cooking so much better.

I play football on a team with my friends and our home ground is just next to the allotment. After training sessions we gather for a beer and a chat in the garden. In the summer I often invite friends to barbecue and hang out here. My mother also uses the allotment as a place to meet with her friends. They sit in the sun, knitting and talking, *hygg*-ing together. 99

Cornelius Simonsen, Vesterbro

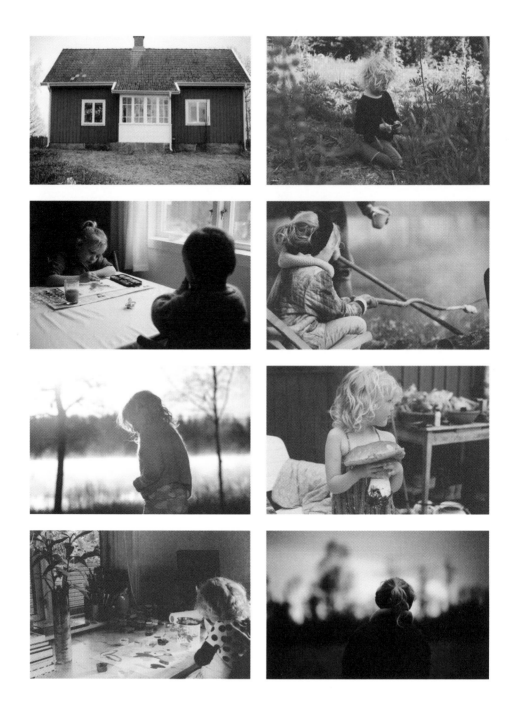

Swedish Farm House

66 We visit our family's house in southern Sweden, only a few hours' drive from Copenhagen, as often as possible. It's like going back in time with no electricity, no running water or internet. It's hidden deep in the forest right next to the most beautiful lake. The fireplace is always lit in the winter to keep us warm and when the sun has gone down you light up candles to read, to play games and even to brush your teeth. To me, nothing is as *hyggelig* as that place, because it makes me feel like I've got all the time in the world. 99

Nanna Mosegaard, Copenhagen

Hygge Is Found
All Over the World

Hicham Bennani is forty years old and lives in the northern part of Jutland with his nine-year-old son, his Danish wife, Satie, and their little newborn baby. He originates from Morocco, where he was born in 1976. At the age of seventeen he moved to England with his family and lived in Brighton for twelve years. For the last eleven years he has lived in Denmark and according to Hicham, *hygge* can be found all over the world, as long as there is togetherness, something for the senses and a feeling of spontaneity.

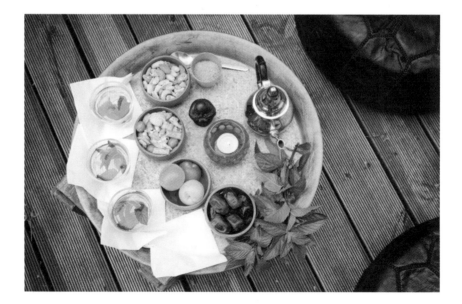

❝ In Morocco, the symbol of hygge is the tray with the mint teapot and the glasses. Before anything gets done, you get together and drink a glass of tea. Usually there are pouffes and cushions to help you chill and loosen up. Some will be dressed in their djellaba and fruit and salted snacks will be served and there will be non-stop talking. Maybe the topic of conversation is something big in the news, something huge overseas, or something that happened in Casablanca. But usually it starts with small talk: 'Have you heard what Fatima did, oh, she got married . . . Really, the daughter of . . .' and then it goes on.

In England I often experienced *hygge* in the pubs. You can 'belong' to a bar, by having your own pewter beer tankard, with your name engraved on it. Here you get together, leave the formal tone outside, joke and talk about issues in a light-hearted way. I especially miss the Sunday pub. In Brighton where my family lived, we used to go for a Sunday pub lunch, where you sit down, have roast lamb and Yorkshire pudding and exchange stories from the weekend. Most stories have been told before, but they are brought up again, as they keep making us laugh, and it all adds to the *hyggelig*, light and relaxed atmosphere.

In the Danish *hygge* you are quite straight with each other and get quickly into the deeper layers of what you really wish to talk about. In Denmark, *hygge* is closely connected to time spent with family and good friends, whereas in Morocco it is more common to *hygge* with people you don't know that well. The intimate space of the home is more open to neighbours and other people you are not that close to.

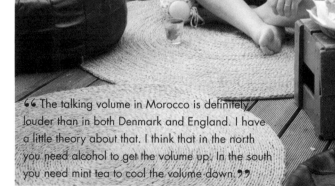

66 The talking volume in Morocco is definitely
louder than in both Denmark and England. I have
a little theory about that. I think that in the north
you need alcohol to get the volume up. In the south
you need mint tea to cool the volume down. 99

The main difference between the Danish *hygge* and the *hygge* I have found in other places is that the Danes have a word for it. Now, living in Denmark and having a word for it makes me more aware of where I find *hygge* and how I bring it into a situation. The word '*hygge*' covers it all – the togetherness, the little something for the senses, and the spontaneity. Having a word for it expresses something quite advanced in a way. When you make a word, that allocates it all in one, it means you are pretty close to the essence of what *hygge* is about.

In my opinion *hygge* can be found all over the world, and there are more similarities than differences. The main value in the universal *hygge* is the fact that in a *hyggelig* atmosphere you can relax and be who you are without meeting judgement.

Actually, *hygge* should be a religion.**99**

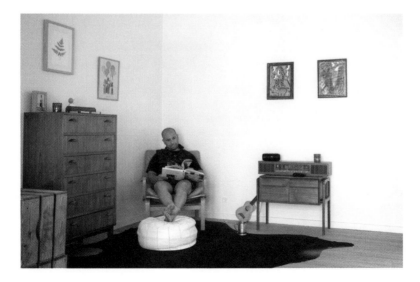

THE POTENTIAL

IN *HYGGE*

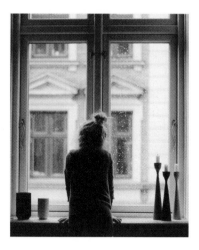

The Danish *hygge* has been criticized politically from both the right and left wing in Denmark.

The left wing criticizes *hygge* for being alienating, introvert and fearful of cultures different from the Scandinavian. The right wing criticizes *hygge* for being a barrier to ambition, intensity and growth. If we *hygge* too much it is bad for productivity, effectiveness and development, they argue.

But there is potential in the core values of *hygge* according to the twenty-five-year-old entrepreneur and folk high school teacher Mikkel Vinther. The Danish Ministry of Culture has asked a number of Danes – including Mikkel Vinther – to put forward their views on Danish culture, and to identify which elements could qualify for a place on UNESCO's list of intangible culture heritage. A list that accepts cultural phenomena such as customs, traditions and knowledge of crafts. And maybe *hygge*. Which is what Mikkel Vinther is keen to see happen.

❝ *Hygge* is when we say: 'There is no discussing politics now – now we are going to *hygge*.' It is when we put aside our differences and cooperate. *Hygge* is where we meet each other as fellow human beings rather than as opposites, and this is where we recognize that we are all in the same boat. *Hygge*, therefore, is a kind of anti-competitiveness.

I would argue that *hygge* as anti-competitiveness has been, in our world view, the basis for characteristic Danish societal movements such as the folk high school movement, the cooperative movement and our strong Danish volunteer culture.

The folk high school movement in Denmark established contemporary learning centres for adults, where the rural population in particular was 'enlightened and enlivened'. The idea behind the folk high school was that students and teachers already came with their own skills and, therefore, each individual always had something to contribute to the community, and everyone has something they would like to be better at. A spell at a folk high school is about finding the desire for learning. There are no exams or grades, and so there is little internal competition. Students as well as teachers enter into new communities, come up with new ideas and create a more community-orientated society – to the benefit of both society and the individual.

One idea stemming from the communal thinking of the folk high school was the cooperative movement. Here, those in agriculture, in particular, stood together firmly against a price-squeezing external market. And instead of entering internal price wars, important, widespread decisions were taken in local areas to start a *joint movement* where all farmers, dairymen and grocers could have *a share* – with a corresponding share from the profits.

Both societal movements are examples of how hygge as anti-competitiveness made community and local areas stronger in Denmark.

And, I believe, the world needs *hygge* – as an antidote to polarization. We need *hygge* to put a lid on all our differences and focus on the enormous set of common values that all people have. Just like the folk high school and the cooperative movement.

Unfortunately, *hygge* 'works' best in homogeneous groups – like the Danish population in the late 1800s – and, therefore, it can sometimes be perceived as introverted and exclusionary. The world needs '*Hygge* 2.0', which not only bears all of *hygge*'s positive values, but which is also outgoing, open and inclusive. *Hygge* creates a breeding ground for fellowship, cooperation and love – values, I believe, every person can agree upon.**"**

How Does *Hygge* Thrive Today?

Hygge is thriving in today's Denmark but is threatened by health ideals, digital media and society's demands for efficiency. If *hygge* is to maintain its position as a favourite pursuit of the Danes, it must rethink itself, according to a leading lifestyle expert, Anne Glad. She says:

❝ *Hygge* thrives and will always have good and favourable conditions in Denmark. The dark time is an eternal valid basis for *hygge*. This is where Danes snuggle up indoors and invite guests over. The home is *hygge*'s cathedral, and it has been for thousands of years. Even the Vikings invited guests to feast in winter, where they enjoyed the *hygge* and planned summer trips. It is that basic home culture that the Danes have continued until today.

Conditions for *hygge* are particularly good during times of economic crises. Due to the recent crisis, our lifestyles have become more introspective, and Danes have spent more time at home. We have become closer in our families and with close friends. We have lit fires in our hearths, we have something simmering on the hob and we have taken out the board games. There is more space for reflection. Instead of it being smart to own something, it has become smart to know something. Therefore we are reading more books, taking courses and attending more lectures in times of crisis. It has also become prestigious to accept positions of trust within the local community, such as on a kindergarten committee, whereas in times of economic growth the classic prestige committee post was outside of familial obligations.

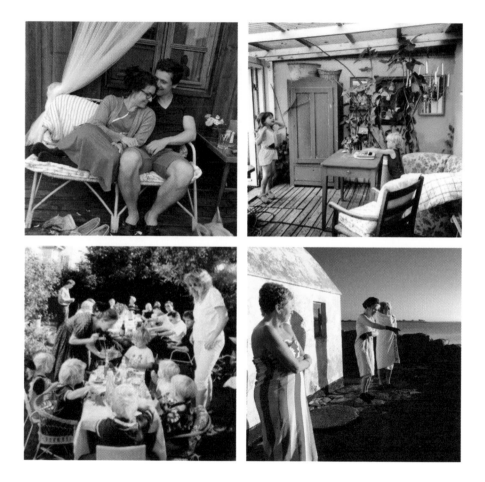

But there are trends in today's society that threaten *hygge*. The enthusiastic worship of the body and health in some parts of the population threatens those joys, which are often associated with foods such as sweets, cakes, beer and wine. The number of fitness centres is increasing, Danes are measuring their blood pressures and cholesterol levels like never before, and thousands are suddenly running marathons; a niche sport that was reserved for a few eager fools in the old days and was never intended to become a popular sport. Seen in this light, *hygge* has a serious image problem, and if the health wave continues to roar and hits the broader population, *hygge* will face an uphill struggle.

Digital and social media are also a threat. Studies show that a large number of Danish families have experienced feeling stressed at times. But Danish parents are not working longer hours, and the amount of leisure time is also the same. What has changed is the number of hours we are spending on digital media, and then, in turn, our need for individualization. It is not enough to be a good citizen who pays their taxes and behaves well; no, we have to have a career, a family, a beautiful home, care for our personal appearance, realize ourselves – and talk about it on social media. These media take time away from time that could be spent together as a family, are disruptive to the presence of our children and can be sources of conflict if parents try to set limits on each other's and their children's use of them.

The good, old-fashioned television is not without its problems, because we risk not being aware of the *hygge* at all when the TV is just blabbering away. Our main components for *hygge* involve bringing family members and sweets together, but when Friday's entertainment rolls across the screen, we gorge on sweets without tasting them and we forget to be present with those we are sitting beside on the sofa. Moreover, it is widely believed that a sneak peek at Facebook is allowed when the TV screen is turned on.

To conquer these threats and retain its popularity with the healthy, modern individual, *hygge* needs to rethink itself. *Hygge* can give us community, presence, contemplation and rest. It can do all this, which is the new luxury; that which we spend so much money on achieving through hiking and yoga holidays – but it needs to get itself off the sofa more often and go out into the fresh air. *Hygge* needs to be something that is done when standing, walking and conversing. *Hygge* needs to be *active* rather than *passive*. *Hygge* is being with the kids in the forest. Walking in a child's footsteps and taking the time to cultivate microscopic experiences like watching a beetle walking across a leaf. *Hygge* needs to convince us that it will follow us if we take the freshly baked rolls outside for a picnic instead of taking them over to the sofa.

Hygge needs to ally itself with some of the new players in the market such as audio products of all kinds. Sales of audio books have just overtaken the sales of e-books. Podcasts and radio programmes are becoming more and more popular. Listening to something instead of taking in knowledge and entertainment visually demands more presence, and that means better conditions for *hygge*.

Most importantly, *hygge* needs to stand tall and remember its history. *Hygge* is the cool thing about being Scandinavian. It is the reason we have a home life that includes others, and not just ourselves. It is the reason why people get together and talk in relaxed and informal gatherings and it is the light in the darkness, which carries us through six cold winter months, and it has done so for more than a thousand years.❞

POSTSCRIPT

Hygge moments are the small everyday moments that make you happy.

The best of them are bright and shining like stars.

Having a word for it makes you aware that they are right in front of your eyes.

Ready for you to collect.

HYGGE DICTIONARY

Baggrundshygge (background-*hygge*). Can be *hygge* music playing in the background, children playing, birds singing, guests chatting and laughing or other *hygge* things going on in the background.

Caféhygge (café-*hygge*). Spending a *hyggelig* time *hygg*-ing in a *hyggelig* café.

Familiehygge (family-*hygge*). E.g. 'Let's have some family-*hygge* on Saturday.' This implies playing a game, making delicious food together. Basically just enjoying family togetherness in whatever form you find *hyggelig*.

Filmhygge (you guessed it: film-*hygge*). *Hygg*-ing while watching a film, e.g. 'Let's have a film-*hygge* evening, Mogens.'

Fødselsdagshygge (birthday-*hygge*). Homemade buns and presents in bed, Danish layer cake (special birthday tradition in Denmark), being with friends celebrating your birthday just the way you like. That is birthday-*hygge*.

Forårshygge (spring-*hygge*), also *sommerhygge* (summer-*hygge*) and *efterårshygge* (autumn-*hygge*). Seasonal *hygge*-words which define different ways of *hygg*-ing depending on the season.

Fredagshygge (Friday-*hygge*), also *Lørdagshygge*
(Saturday-*hygge*), *Søndagshygge* (Sunday-*hygge*).
Popular *hygge* words, and all good days for *hygge*
time. *Hygge* is a time off from work thing.

Halvhyggeligt (half-*hygge*). Used to describe an
unsuccessful family dinner or other kind of *hygge*
arrangement, e.g. 'How was the dinner, love?' 'Oh, it
was half *hyggelig*.'

Hjemmehygge (homely-*hygge*). E.g. 'What are you doing
tonight, Anne-Dorthe?' 'Oh, we are just having a
hjemmehyggeaften' (a homely *hygge* evening).
Meaning, we are staying home to *hygge*, instead of
going out to *hygge*.

Hyggeaften (*hygge*-evening). Practically, a *hyggeaften*
implies eating *hygge*-food and spending *hygge*-time
with loved ones. Often used about an evening where
you stay home to *hygge* instead of going out. A
hyggeaften is spent watching a film while eating
hygge-snacks, or playing a game, having a glass of
wine, or just *hygge*-talking. See *Hjemmehygge*.

Hyggebajer (*hygge*-beer). A beer you drink when you want
to have *bajerhygge* – *hygge* with beer, e.g. 'Henning,
let's have a *hygge*-beer.'

Hyggebamse (*hygge*-teddy). E.g. 'Did you remember to
bring your *hygge*-teddy bear, Sofus?'

Hyggebelysning (*hygge*-lighting). E.g. 'Look, Sigrid, this restaurant looks nice.' 'Oh no, Bjarke, the light here is too bright. Why don't they have *hygge*-lighting instead? It would be so much better for the atmosphere.' (Go to p.133 to find out how to make your *hygge*-lighting.)

Hyggebinge (*hygge*-binge-watch). E.g. 'Louise is *hygge*-binging the first season of *Skam* on NRK.'

Hyggebold (*hygge*-ball). Slang for a game of football played for the sake of *hygge*. People are into *hygge*-ball to have a *hyggelig* time playing, and not necessarily to win. It might not even imply a game. *Hygge*-ball can simply be kicking the ball around in a circle, doing some *hyggelig* tricks (not too fancy tricks though . . .).

Hyggedag (*hygge*-day). E.g. 'Steffen, let's skip school today and have a *hygge*-day instead.'

Hyggefacade (*hygge*-facade). *Hygge*-facade is a mask you put on in a social context to pretend that there is *hygge* going on, when in fact it isn't *hyggelig* at all. This is done to avoid a conflict or being dramatic, just to hang in there – putting on the *hygge*-facade until it is time to go home.

Hyggefiskeri (*hygge*-fishing). Going fishing to have a *hyggelig* time, e.g. 'What are you doing today, Arne?' 'I am going *hygge*-fishing.'

Hyggehejsa (a greeting or farewell, like 'toodle-oo'). Say it to your friends when you say hello or goodbye, but be aware that it is a very fresh, informal and happy greeting – so perhaps don't greet your boss this way.

Hyggehjørne (*hygge*-corner). *Hygge* happens a lot in corners, e.g. 'What a beautiful armchair, Dorrit.' 'Thank you, Hanne, I think I will use it in my *hygge*-corner.'

Hyggejam (*hygge*-jamming). Playing music in order to *hygge* – and just jamming. 'Come on, guys, you wanna *hyggejam?*'

Hyggekrog (*hygge*-nook). E.g. 'Oh, Astrid, what a *hygge*-nook you've got there. I bet you spend a lot of time *hygg*-ing there.'

Hyggekryds (*hygge*-crossword). Solving crossword puzzles for the sake of *hygge*, e.g. 'I am just sitting here with my *hygge*-crossword.'

Hyggelæsning (*hygge*-reading). Reading as part of a *hygge*-moment.

Hyggeland (*hygge*-country). Nickname for Denmark. 'Denmark, you *hygge*-country.'

Hyggelig (*hygge*, adjective). A bit like cosy, e.g. 'What a *hyggelig* café, Hans.' Or 'It was so *hyggelig* to see you, Lise.' Pronounced *hygge*-lee. Forms: *hyggelig*, *hyggeligere*, *hyggeligst* (*hyggelig*, more *hyggelig*, most *hyggelig*).

Hyggemad (*hygge*-food). E.g. 'Children, what do you want for dinner?' 'I want *hygge*-food!' See 'Inviting *Hygge* to the Table' chapter for good *hygge*-food.

Hyggemennesker (*hygge*-people). Meaning people who are seriously into *hygge*. 'Kirsten and Henrik are some really sweet *hygge*-people we spend lots of time with.'

Hyggemiddag (*hygge*-dinner). E.g. 'Let's have a *hyggemiddag* soon, Birgit.' Something you invite your friends to. Either gather a lot of friends, or just invite a handful. The more people, the bigger the *hygge*.

Hyggemøbler (*hygge*-furniture). *Hygge*-furniture is furniture that invites you to *hygge* in it.

Hyggemor (*hygge*-mother). A woman who is good at *hygg*-ing around other people in a caring and loving way, like a mother, e.g. 'Mona is our *hygge*-mother at the after-school care.'

Hyggemotionist (*hygge*-exerciser/jogger/person who works out). When adding *hygge* it implies that the person exercises slowly, mostly for the *hygge*, and not really to get in better shape, more to have a good time – perhaps with a friend. 'Grethe, yes – she sure is a *hygge*-exerciser.'

Hyggen (THE *hygge*). Use this form when talking about a specified *hygge* going on, e.g. 'The *hyggen* at grandma's place was superb.'

Hyggenygge (seriously good *hygge*). '*Nygge*' isn't really a word but just rhymes with *hygge*, a bit like saying something meaningless like 'cosy-wosy'. But also used ironically – 'Oh, so you're *hyggenygging*.' Using *hyggenygge* this way is an insult or a critique on the *hygge*.

Hyggeonkel (*hygge*-uncle) and ***Hyggetante*** (*hygge*-aunt). Not necessarily biologically speaking, but perhaps a friend of the family who is good at playing and being around kids. It is also used about people who are really good at *hygg*-ing around other people, making a good atmosphere, baking cakes, inviting people home to *hygge*, always being jolly and nice. (see **Hygge om**, p.12).

Hyggepianist (*hygge*-pianist). A pianist playing to make a *hygge* atmosphere, e.g. 'There was an amazing atmosphere there, right, Thor?' 'Yes, they even had a *hygge*-pianist.'

Hyggerum (*hygge*-room). E.g. a living room with a *hygge*-sofa or a *hygge*-mattress that invites you to *hygge* in.

Hyggesludder (*hygge*-chat). E.g. 'I met Lotte in the bakery and we had a *hygge*-chat. We just talked about all the things that are going on in the neighbourhood.'

Hyggesnak (*hygge*-talk). Where *sludder* is more implying a chat about all and nothing, *snak* is more substantial, e.g. 'It was so nice to see Sofie the other day. We *hygge*-talked until three in the morning.'

Hyggespreder (*hygge*-spreader). Used about a *hyggelig* person who is really good at spreading *hygge* to people around them. It is also used ironically for letting out a fart in a social context, and 'spreading *hygge*' while being among other people.

Hyggestemning (*hygge*-atmosphere). E.g. 'We went to a new café yesterday. There was such a good *hygge*-atmosphere.'

Hyggestund (*hygge*-moment). E.g. 'We just enjoyed a *hygge*-moment together in the sun.' Good photos capture this special moment. Not just the aesthetics of it, but the entire atmosphere around the *hygge*-moment.

Hyggesyg (*hygge*-sickness). Having to stay home from work, but not so sick that you have to lie down in pain all day. So, walking around at home, with a scarf, slippers and warm socks on, and watching films and eating nice things – but not well enough to go to work.

Hyggetempo (*hygge*-pace). A day in *hyggetempo* is a Saturday with nothing to do. A run in *hyggetempo* is something you do just for the *hygge* sake of it.

Hyggetime (*hygge*-hour). Especially used in schools about a lesson with no teaching – just *hygge*. Probably some drawing, reading aloud and eating cake.

Hyggetur (*hygge*-trip). E.g. a trip to the forest or the beach together with someone for the sake of *hygge* – 'Let's go on a *hygge*-trip together, Emil.'

Jordbærhygge (strawberry-*hygge*). A very Danish kind of *hygge* in the summer is eating, buying or collecting strawberries. It is closely connected to memories and traditions with strawberries, which makes it *hyggelig*.

Julehygge (Christmas-*hygge*). As we all know it, with traditions, great Christmas food, lights decorating the streets, *hygge*-atmosphere everywhere. And of course having *hygge*-moments with your family and loved ones.

Landsbyhygge (village-*hygge*). Very common form of *hygge*, because of the great amount of *hygge* in small villages.

Morgenhygge (morning-*hygge*). Probably strolling around the house in slippers, low tempo, loads of time. Or waking up with someone you love and having a *hyggelig* time in one way or another before the day really begins.

Morgenmadshygge (breakfast-*hygge*). An important part of Saturday and Sunday morning. Perhaps a brunch if you wake up late. Involves all your favourite breakfast things, a newspaper, time to relax and a nice cuppa.

Nissehygge (gnome-*hygge*). A Christmas thing, connected to all the things a gnome does in Danish Christmas traditions: they eat porridge in the attic, tease you in a *hyggelig* way, live in small and *hyggelig* places in your house. Gnome-*hygge* is also decorating the house with gnomes for Christmas and thereby creating gnome-*hygge* and Christmas-*hygge*.

Øhygge (island-*hygge*). There can be so much *hygge* on Danish islands. Samsø, Bornholm, Fanø, Anholt, Ærø and Langeland are a few of the many *hygge* islands in Denmark with loads of island-*hygge*.

Ølhygge (beer-*hygge*). Some would say a very Danish thing. A Carlsberg in one hand, sitting in the sun after work is beer-*hygge*. Or just celebrating that you are off from work by enjoying a beer. Can also imply getting drunk in a *hyggelig* way with friends.

Pigehygge (girl-*hygge*). Like girl power, just in a *hyggelig* way. Girls being together doing all kinds of *hyggelig* stuff. Talking and being girly in a very *hyggelig* way.

Råhygge (raw-*hygge*). *Hygge* in its purest form, e.g. 'It was totally raw-*hygge*.'

Tehygge (tea-*hygge*). *Hygg*-ing with tea.

Uhygge (un-*hygge*). Used when speaking about a dismal or sinister atmosphere, horror. Or as *uhyggelig* (adj.) – cheerless, comfortless, scary or spooky. The absolute opposite of *hygge*!

Vinterhygge (winter-*hygge*). Winther-*hygge* is keeping warm when it's cold and dark outside, lighting a candle and having a *hyggelig* time. Winter-*hygge* can also be looking at a landscape with beautiful snow that makes the atmosphere *hyggelig*. And then you say 'That's sheer winter-*hygge*.'

Vovsehygge (dog-*hygge*). *Hygge* in company with a dog, e.g. 'We had a day full of doggy-*hygge*'.

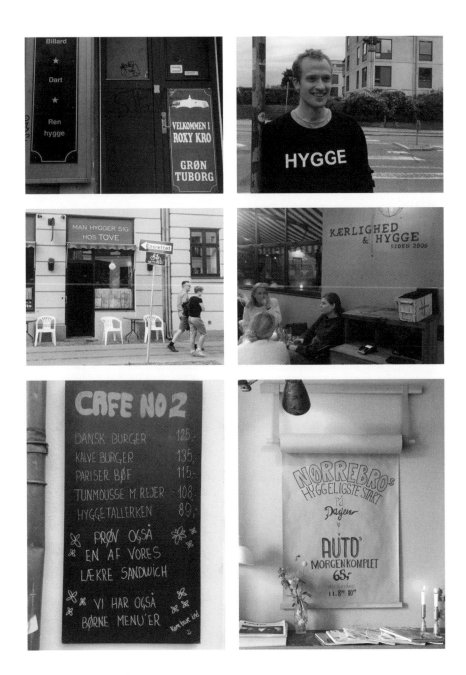

When you take a look at these *hygge*-words in Danish it is clear that there are more words where *hygge* is the first word in the compound, e.g. *hygge*-food, *hygge*-weather. And fewer words where *hygge* is the last word, e.g. raw-*hygge*, family-*hygge*. All the words have this in common; they tell us something about the things we do together – talk, eat, drink – togetherness things. The words are often used to describe specific times, occasions and circumstances – Christmas, evening, summer, autumn, Friday, morning, Easter and so on. But no matter what kind of *hygge*-word we are talking about, they all share the same essence – *hygge* implies something that is relaxing, enjoyable, loveable and charming, and something we do together.

Make Your Own *Hygge*-Words

You can easily make your own *hygge*-words – just find a word and start or end it with *hygge*. Think about what is *hyggelig* – buns, music, candy, candles, a bonfire, pillows, blankets, the weekend – and add *hygge*: *hygge*-buns, *hygge*-music, *hygge*-candy, bonfire-*hygge*, *hygge*-pillows, *hygge*-blanket and the *hygge*-weekend. It's really easy and there are so many combinations. If you find *hygge* somewhere, you are, without a doubt, allowed to create a word that describes it. It can be untraditional – a ride on the bus can become a *hygge*-bus ride, if it is a *hyggelig* one. A need for *hygge* can become a *hygge*-need. *Hyggelig* shopping can become *hygge*-shopping. Or even a meeting at work can become a *hygge*-meeting, if it is *hyggelig* enough to not feel like work. Don't hold back – go all in with the *hygge*-words.

INSPIRATION

Scandinavian Interior Design

These are Danish magazines with great inspirational material. Some are more *hyggelig* than others, but all of them are good, magazine-wise. You can find most of them in the app store on your smartphone, and even though they are in Danish the pictures are very inspiring.

- *Alt for damerne interiør*
- *Boligmagasinet*
- *Bo bedre*
- *Boligliv*

For different kinds of inspiration, you could also try:

- Watching films and having a look at great scenography and production design
- *Christiania Interiør – Interior* by Karina Tengberg and Tami Christiansen (Copenhagen, Nyt Nordisk Forlag, 2011)
- *Kunsthåndværkerhjem* by Anitta Behrendt, Christiana B. Kjeldsen and Rikke Graff Juel (Aarhus, Turbine, 2016)
- *The Kinfolk Home* by Nathan Williams (New York, Artisan Books, 2015)
- *The Life-Changing Magic of Tidying* by Marie Kondo, (London, Vermilion, 2014)

- *A Perfectly Kept House is a Sign of a Misspent Life* by Mary Randolph Carter (New York, Rizzoli International Publications, 2010)
- *The Danish Way of Parenting – A Guide to Raising the Happiest Children in the World* by Jessica Alexander and Iben Sandahl (Copenhagen, Ehrhorn Hummerston, 2014)
- Homesick DIY on homesick.nu

Food

Cook Scandinavian by Camilla Plum (London, Kyle Books, 2015)

GRØD Kogebogen (English version) by Lasse Skjønning Andersen (Copenhagen, Vandkunsten, 2015)

The Nordic Kitchen: One Year of Family Cooking by Claus Meyer (London, Mitchell Beazley, 2016)

The Green Kitchen: Delicious and Healthy Vegetarian Recipes for Every Day by Luise Vindahl and David Frenkiel (Stockholm, Hardie Grant Books, 2013)

Everyday Super Food by Jamie Oliver (London, Michael Joseph, 2015)

The Kinfolk Table by Nathan William (New York, Artisan, 2013)

Instagram inspiration list

@margrethesa / @nannamosegaard / @amalielaulundtrudsoe @louisise / @chrisbk79 / @miastensgaard / @rosacelinderfaurholm / @neelronholt / @luisegreenkitchenstories / @gkstories / @homesickblog

Acknowledgements

This book was created with help from all these wonderful people and their perspectives on hygge.

Ditte Lysgaard for a lot of good hours on the high way and an equal lot of beautiful photos for the book.

Thank you Júlia Reig, Cornelius Simonsen, Neel Rønholt, Fanny Bruun Andersen, Anna Elisabeth Gonge, Vibeke Gonge, Marendine Ladegaard and friends, Niels Erling, Sara Andersen, Lea Sommer, Grete Petersen, Jakob Nyholm Jessen and Signe Fog Christensen, Agnes and Niels, Ole Viby, Louise B. Kjeldsen, Palle Fogh, Ina Schack Vestergaard and family, Christina B. Kjeldsen, Hicham Bennani and Satie Espersen, Lennart Lajboschitz and Absalon, Amalie Laulund Trudsø, Søren from pub "90'eren", Nanna Mosegaard, Margrethe Sønderlund Andersen, Edith Fogh Vindelev, Tilde Vindelev Vengsgaard, Kirstine Fogh Vindelev and Carmen for being the best everyday *hygge* experts.

Mikkel Vinther, Iben Sandahl, Anne Glad, Heidi Boye, Marie Stender, Mads Olsen, Master Fatman, Asger Bay Christiansen, Jørgen og Flora Melchiorsen, Signe Bindslev Hansen and Peter Bundgaard Rützou, Heidi Schiøtz, Christian Bjørnskov, Jeppe Gjervig Gram and Mia Stensgaard for your expertise that put *hygge* into a greater perspective.

Michelle Kristensen, Camilla Plum and Lasse Skjønning Andersen for generously sharing your *hyggeligste* recipes.

Camilla Marie, Tatiana & Mette from Homesick for making wonderfully inspiring do-it-yourself recipes.

Amalie Laulund Trudsø and Rosinante for lending us a bit of *Summerhouse*.

Sinéad Quirke Køngerskov for skilfully translating material from Danish to English.

Margrethe Sønderlund Andersen and Nanna Mosegaard – and your families for sharing and being able to capture the true hygge moments so brilliantly.

Thank you Rosa and Mikkel Celinder Faurholm, Lulu Betz, Magnus Lindeberg, Louise B.Kjeldsen, Amalie Laulund Trudsø, Jon and Gigger Agger Jørgensen, Neel Rønholt, Mikkala Kissi, Martin Pedersen and the boys, Tilde Vindelev Vengsgaard, Tone Mygind Rostbøll, Christina B. Kjeldsen, Susanne Klixbüll, Rolf Konow, Per Arnesen, Anders Heinrichsen, Ida Marie Winge Café Auto and Catarina Nedertoft Jessen for sharing your wonderful photos in the book.

Christina B. Kjeldsen, for immense help and comforting advice when we had trouble seeing the forest for the trees.

Jeppe Trolle Linnet, for being a very hyggelig and excellent hygge-expert and sparring partner.

Fiona Crosby for your great patience, trust, encouragement and expertise. Karen Bryden and Sophie Elletson for being indispensable in this process.

Louise Moore and John Bond – this book wouldn't have happened if it wasn't for you two and the lovely days we spent together.

Torkild Fogh Vindelev who has untiringly been a loyal and personal co-editor, Mathias Sommer for sharp and professional feedback and Sine Bach Jakobsen for a skilled read-through.

Family, friends and great colleagues for being inspiring and teaching me the importance of *hygge*.

And thank you Kirsten Højte, Henning Lynggaard, Marie Højte Lynggaard, Mathias Sommer, and Lise Søderberg, Peter Tourell, Tine Tourell Søderberg and Torkild Fogh Vindelev for a life full of hygge, love and support.

Sources

Danmark in numbers 2016, Danmarks Statistik • En fortælling om Danmark i det 20. arhundrede, Bo Lidegaard, 2011, Gyldendal • Politikens Danmarkshistorie 2007 • Man har et standpunkt, Niels Krause Kjær • denstoredanske. dk • danmarkshistorien.dk by Aarhus University • Money can't buy me Hygge, Jeppe Trolle Linnet, 2009 • Cozy Interiority, Jeppe Trolle Linnet, 2014 • Fødevarer og Sundhed i senmodernismen: En indsigt i hyggefænomenet og de relaterede fødevarepraksiser, Heidi Boye, 2010 • Romerriget, Radio 24syv, programme week 52, 2012 • Elsk dit hjem fra a-å, by Ranvita La Cour, Nyt Nordisk forlag Arnold Busck (2009) • ordnet.dk • Den undertrykkende danske hygge, Kristeligt Dagblad september 12th 2014 • Levende lys er hurtig hygge, Politiken, September 27th, 2015 • Forsker søger ind til hyggens væsen, Vagn Erik Andersen, Magazine Ny Viden, SDU • Hyggeforsker: Danskere med og uden penge hygger sig forskelligt, Politiken, Helle Lorenzen, 2013 • Hygge er ærligt, usmart og ærkedansk, Kristeligt Dagblad, 2009 • Nu skal vi rigtig hygge os . Weekendavisen, September 11th 2015 • Sådan opdrager vi børn til at blive lykkelige, Kristeligt dagblad December 17th 2015 • Vi bliver snart verdensmestre i slik, Politiken, march 2nd 2015 • Get cosy: why we should all embrace the Danish art of 'hygge', the Telegraph, 15th of October, 2015 • Scandi-Mania documentary, with Hugh Fearnley-Whittingstall, 2014 • Ud og Se Magazine, March 2016 • The human animal, BBC documentary, Desmond Morris • Hygge som våben mod terror, Rune Lykkeberg, Politiken, February 21st 2015 • Rapport: Danskernes forbrug af stearinlys, Boluis, nov. 2014

Credits

p4: Marie © *Anders Heinrichsen* • **p7:** Clockwise from top left: six-year-old Marie with her younger sister Tine, Marie's boyfriend Torkild Fogh Vindelev, friends from High School © Fanny Bruun Andersen, and Marie with her mother Lise Søderberg (family photos) • **p11:** Family photos © Margrethe Sønderlund Andersen, Nanna Mosegaard and Rosa Celinder Faurholm • **p20:** Seasons © Christina B. Kjeldsen and Amalie Laulund Trudsø • **p23:** Landscapes © Christina B. Kjeldsen • **p24:** Friends camping in Sweden © Martin Pedersen • **p26:** Sunset on the terrace © Margrethe Sønderlund Andersen • **p31:** Clockwise from top left: Marie's childhood friends Josephine Fayard and Anna Katrine Waage, Marie and her father, a true hygge moment, Marie's sister and best friend Tine (family photos), film set of *Sofa* © Anna Emma Haudal, film set of 1864 © Per Arnesen, Rosa and her son Isak, favourite childhood climbing tree (family photos) • **p32:** Ingeborg and Holger playing in a glade © Margrethe Sønderlund Andersen • **p34:** A winter evening around the fire © Margrethe Sønderlund Andersen • **pp36-39:** Marendine Krainert Ladegaard having a hyggelig evening with friends and colleagues © Ditte Lysgaard Holm • **pp40-43:** Anna Elisabeth Gonge at home in Jutland © Ditte Lysgaard Holm • **p44:** From top: Theodor and Sonja reading a bedtime story © Tone Rostbøll Mygind, family time on the beach and in the garden house © Margrethe Sønderlund Andersen • **p50:** Nora in the Swedish farm house © Nanna Mosegaard • **p50:** From top: Morten and Holger on an evening walk © Margrethe Sønderlund Andersen, Theodor and Sonja and their father © Tone Rostbøll Mygind, Alfred and Uffe reading © Christina B. Kjeldsen • **pp56-60:** Lea Sommer and her grandmother Grete Petersen at Grete's home in Odense © Ditte Lysgaard Holm • **pp62-63:** An everyday night in the 1916 Copenhagen pub Vinstue 90 © Ditte Lysgaard Holm • **pp64-65:** Dining in the community centre Absalon in Copenhagen © Ditte Lysgaard Holm • **p70:** From left: Elsa and Isac in the kitchen © David Frenkiel at Green Kitchen Stories, picnic, freshly-picked strawberries and dinner preparations © Margrethe Sønderlund Andersen • **pp74-77:** Ina's kitchen © Ditte Lysgaard Holm • **pp 80-83:** Palle's kitchen © Ditte Lysgaard Holm • **pp86–89:** Louise's Potato Sandwiches © Ditte Lysgaard Holm • **p90:** Rødgrød med fløde from Lise Søderberg's kitchen © Marie Tourell Søderberg • **p92:** Lasse Skjønning Andersen's favourite porridge © Chris Tonnesen • **p94:** Snobrød in the making © Lise Søderberg • **p96:** Traditional layer cake with freshly-picked berries © Louise B. Kjeldsen • Michelle Kristensen's snickers © Joachim Wichmann • **p101:** Open air wedding, Apple Flower Festival on Lilleø arranged by the Danish chef Claus Meyer © Kim Tonning • **p104-107:** Jakob Nyholm Jessen and Signe Fog Christensen with their children Agnes and Niels at home in Sealand © Ditte Lysgaard Holm • Ingeborg's reading hyggespot © Margrethe Sønderlund Andersen • **p111:** A personal home © Karina Tengberg • **p113:** PH-lamp in a kitchen in Frederiksberg © Jon and Gigger Agger Jørgensen • **p114:** Summerhouse in Northern Sealand © Magnus Lindeberg • **p117:** Hallway © Peter Kragballe • **p119:** Kitchen © Karina Tengberg • **p121:** Living room © Peter Kragballe • **p123:** Bathroom © Yvonne Wilhelmsen • **p125:** Bedroom © Peter Kragballe • **p126:** Ready for water colour painting © Tilde Vindelev Vengsgaard • **p128:** From left: Flowers from the garden © Margrethe Sønderlund Andersen, Field flowers © Neel Rønholt, Cotton branch © Nanna Mosegaard • **p129, 130:** Plants, Corners © Karina Tengberg • **p131:** Presents and heirlooms © Peter Kragballe • **p132:** From top: Lighting up the garden house © Margrethe Sønderlund Andersen, An evening at Café Auto in Copenhagen © Café Auto, Looking in © Nanna Mosegaard • **p135:** From top: Candle © Marie Tourell Søderberg, Getting ready for Christmas Eve © Nanna Mosegaard, Painting stones from the beach © Margrethe Sønderlund Andersen • **p136-137:** Books, Recycle © Peter Kragballe • **p138:** Instruments © Marie Tourell Søderberg • **p140:** Souvenirs © Karina Tengberg • **p141:** Mix and match © Peter Kragballe • **p143:** Workspace © Peter Kragballe • **p144-150:**

Internationally acclaimed restaurant NOMA © Mikkel Heriba • **p152:** Danish actresses Marie Bach Hansen and Trine Dyrholm in the *The Legacy* © Per Arnesen • **p153:** Danish actors Mads Mikkelsen, Søren Malling and Birthe Neumann in the absurd film comedy *Men and Chicken* © Rolf Konow • **p154:** Actress Trine Dyrholm in the TV-series *The Legacy* © Martin Lehmann • **p156:** Behind the scenes of *The Legacy* © Mia Stensgaard • **p160:** Danish nature © Amalie Laulund Trudsø, Nelson L (Flickr) and Christina B. Kjeldsen • **p162-163:** Nora in the evening sun and under the cherry blossom © Nanna Mosegaard • **p165:** Snowdrop letter © Marie Tourell Søderberg • **p166:** Clockwise from top left: Christina Yhman in flower field © Amalie Laulund Trudsø, Nora and friend picking strawberries © Nanna Mosegaard, Berries and sea © Amalie Laulund Trudsø, Sleeping under the sky © Margrethe Sønderlund Andersen • **p168:** Elderflower Cordial © Amalie Laulund Trudsø • **p170:** Apples and bonfires © Margrethe Sønderlund Andersen, Forest © Christina B. Kjeldsen • **p172-174:** Hobby-clay bowl and plank table © Homesick DIY • **p176:** Clockwise from top left: Amalie Laulund Trudsø in Swedish farm house © Louise B. Kjeldsen, Sleighride © Christina B. Kjeldsen, Indoor time © Margrethe Sønderlund Andersen, Homemade Christmas decorations © Amalie Laulund Trudsø, St Lucy's Day © Nanna Mosegård, Snow © Amalie Laulund Trudsø • **p178:** Hygge lights © Homesick DIY • **p181:** Kyndelmisse-girls © Marie Tourell Søderberg • **p182:** Family time in sunset © Margrethe Sønderlund Andersen • **p184:** Reading in the garden house © Margrethe Sønderlund Andersen • **p185:** Extract from Sommerhus © Amalie Laulund Trudsø and Rosinante/Rosinante & Co, Copenhagen 2016. **p186:** Clockwise from top left: Emil Krøll and Mark Hau enjoying a beer © Marie Tourell Søderberg, Allotment in Sydhavnen © Mikkala Kissi, Allotment and garden © Lulu Betz, Allotment in Kløvermarken © Marie Tourell Søderberg • **p188:** A Swedish family farm house © Nanna Mosegaard • **p190-193:** Hicham Bennani at home © Ditte Lysgaard Holm • **p196:** Looking out on the rain in the streets of Copenhagen © Nanna Mosegaard • **p200:** Clockwise from top left: Margrethe Sønderlund Andersen and her husband Morten, Playing in the Garden House © Margrethe Sønderlund Andersen, Ærø Winter bathing club © Catarina Nedertoft Jessen, Birthday dinner in the 90's © Gigger Agger • **p204:** Stars © *Strftime, Flickr* • **p215:** Hygge from differents spots in Denmark, from Faaborg in the South to Copenhagen in the East © Kathrine Højte Lynggaard.